D1216715

Basics of PET Imaging

Physics, Chemistry, and Regulations

Gopal B. Saha, PhD

Department of Molecular and Functional Imaging,
The Cleveland Clinic Foundation, Cleveland, Ohio

Basics of PET Imaging

Physics, Chemistry, and Regulations

With 64 Illustrations

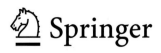
⚘ Springer

Gopal B. Saha, PhD
Department of Molecular and Functional Imaging
The Cleveland Clinic Foundation
Cleveland, OH 44195
USA

Library of Congress Cataloging-in-Publication Data

Saha, Gopal B.
  Basics of PET imaging physics, chemistry, and regulations / Gopal B. Saha.
    p. ; cm.
  Includes bibliographical references and index.
  ISBN 0-387-21307-4 (alk. paper)
  1. Tomography, Emission.   2. Medical physics.
  [DNLM: 1. Tomography, Emission-Computed–methods.   2. Prospective Payment
System.   3. Radiopharmaceuticals.   4. Technology, Radiologic.   5. Tomography,
Emission-Computed–instrumentation. WN 206 S131b 2004]   I. Title.
RC78.7.T62S24 2004
616.07′575—dc22

                                                          2004048107

ISBN 0-387-21307-4   Printed on acid-free paper.

Printed in the United States of America.   (BS/EB)

9 8 7 6 5 4 3 2 1   SPIN 10987100

springeronline.com

*To my
teachers, mentors, and friends*

Preface

From the early 1970s to mid-1990s, positron emission tomography (PET) as a diagnostic imaging modality had been for the most part used in experimental research. Clinical PET started only a decade ago. ^{82}Rb-RbCl and ^{18}F-Fluorodeoxyglucose were approved by the U.S. Food and Drug administration in 1989 and 1994, respectively, for clinical PET imaging. Reimbursement by Medicare was approved in 1995 for ^{82}Rb-PET myocardial perfusion imaging and for ^{18}F-FDG PET for various oncologic indications in 1999. Currently several more PET procedures are covered for reimbursement.

Based on the incentive from reimbursement for PET procedures and accurate and effective diagnosis of various diseases, PET centers are growing in the United States and worldwide. The importance of PET imaging has flourished to such a large extent that the Nuclear Medicine Technology Certification Board (NMTCB) is planning to introduce a PET specialty examination in 2004 for nuclear medicine technologists, as well as an augmented version of the PET specialty examination in 2005 for registered radiographers and radiation therapy technologists. Courses are being offered all over the country to train physicians and technologists in PET technology. Many books on clinical PET have appeared in the market, but no book on the basics of PET imaging is presently available. Obviously, such a book is needed to fulfill the requirements of these courses and certifications.

This book focuses on the fundamentals of PET imaging, namely, physics, instrumentation, production of PET radionuclides and radiopharmaceuticals, and regulations concerning PET. The chapters are concise but comprehensive enough to make the topic easily understandable. Balanced reviews of pertinent basic science information and a list of suggested reading at the end of each chapter make the book an ideal text on PET imaging technology. Appropriate tables and appendixes include data and complement the book as a valuable reference for nuclear medicine professionals such as physicians, residents, and technologists. Technologists and residents taking board examinations would benefit most from this book because of its brevity and clarity of content.

The book contains 11 chapters. The subject of each chapter is covered on a very basic level and in keeping with the objective of the book. It is assumed that the readers have some basic understanding of physics and chemistry available in standard nuclear medicine literature. At the end of each chapter, a set of questions is included to provoke the reader to assess the sufficiency of knowledge gained.

Chapter 1 briefly reviews the structure and nomenclature of the atoms, radioactive decay and related equations, and interaction of radiation with matter. This is the gist of materials available in many standard nuclear medicine physics book. Chapter 2 describes the properties of various detectors used in PET scanners. Descriptions of PET scanners, hybrid scintillation cameras, PET/CT scanners, small animal PET scanners, and mobile PET scanners from different manufacturers as well as their features are given. Chapter 3 details how two-dimensional and three-dimensional data are acquired in PET and PET/CT imaging. Also included are the different factors that affect the acquired data and their correction method. Chapter 4 describes the image reconstruction technique and storage and display of the reconstructed images. A brief reference is made to DICOM, PACS, and teleradiology. The performance characteristics of different PET scanners such as spatial resolution, sensitivity, scatter fraction, and so on, are given in Chapter 5. Quality control tests and acceptance tests of PET scanners are also included. Chapter 6 contains the general description of the principles of cyclotron operation and the production of common PET radionuclides. The synthesis and quality control of some common PET radiopharmaceuticals are described in Chapter 7. Chapter 8 covers pertinent regulations concerning PET imaging. FDA, NRC, DOT, and state regulations are discussed. In Chapter 9, a historical background on reimbursement for PET procedures, and different current codes for billing and the billing process are provided. Chapter 10 outlines a variety of factors that are needed in the design of a new PET center. A cost estimate for setting up a PET facility is presented. Chapter 11 provides protocols for four common PET and PET/CT procedures.

I do not pretend to be infallible in writing a book with such significant scientific information. Errors of both commission and omission may have occurred, and I would appreciate having them brought to my attention by the readers.

I would like to thank the staff in our Department of Molecular and Functional Imaging for their assistance in many forms. I am grateful to Ms. Lisa M. Saake, Director of Healthcare Economics, Tyco Healthcare/Mallinckrodt Medical, for her contribution to Chapter 9 in clarifying several issues regarding reimbursement and reshaping the front part of the chapter.

It is beyond the scope of words to express my gratitude to Mrs. Rita Konyves, who undertook the challenge of typing and retyping the manuscript as much as I did in writing it. Her commitment and meticulous effort in the timely completion of the manuscript deserves nothing but my sincere gratitude and thanks.

I am grateful and thankful to Robert Albano, Senior Clinical Medical Editor, for his suggestion and encouragement to write this book, and others at Springer for their support in publishing it.

Cleveland, OH   *Gopal B. Saha, PhD*

Contents

1
Radioactive Decay and Interaction of Radiation with Matter

Atomic Structure

Matter is composed of atoms. An atom consists of a nucleus containing protons (Z) and neutrons (N), collectively called nucleons, and electrons rotating around the nucleus. The sum of neutrons and protons (total number of nucleons) is the mass number denoted by A. The properties of neutrons, protons, and electrons are listed in Table 1.1. The number of electrons in an atom is equal to the number of protons (atomic number Z) in the nucleus. The electrons rotate along different energy shells designated as K-shell, L-shell, M-shell, etc. (Figure 1-1). Each shell further consists of subshells or orbitals, e.g., the K-shell has s orbital; the L-shell has s and p orbitals; the M-shell has s, p, and d orbitals, and the N-shell has s, p, d, and f orbitals. Each orbital can accommodate only a limited number of electrons. For example, the s orbital contains up to 2 electrons; the p orbital, 6 electrons; the d orbital, 10 electrons; and the f orbital, 14 electrons. The capacity number of electrons in each orbital adds up to give the maximum number of electrons that each energy shell can hold. Thus, the K-shell contains 2 electrons; the L-shell 8 electrons, the M-shell 18 electrons, and so forth.

A unique combination of a given number of protons and neutrons in a nucleus leads to an atom called the nuclide. A nuclide X is represented by $^A_Z X_N$. Some nuclides (270 or so) are stable, while others (more than 2700) are unstable. The unstable nuclides are termed the radionuclides, most of which are artificially produced in the cyclotron or reactor, with a few naturally occurring. The nuclides having the same number of protons are called the isotopes, e.g., $^{12}_6 C$ and $^{14}_6 C$; the nuclides having the same number of neutrons are called the isotones, e.g., $^{16}_8 O_8$ and $^{15}_7 N_8$; the nuclides having the same mass number are called the isobars, e.g., ^{131}I and ^{131}Xe; and the nuclides with the same mass number but differing in energy are called the isomers, e.g., ^{99m}Tc and ^{99}Tc.

This chapter is a brief overview of the materials covered and is written on the assumption that the readers are familiar with the basic concept of these materials.

TABLE 1.1. Characteristics of electrons and nucleons.

Particle	Charge	Mass (amu)[a]	Mass (kg)	Mass (MeV)[b]
Electron	−1	0.000549	0.9108×10^{-30}	0.511
Proton	+1	1.00728	1.6721×10^{-27}	938.78
Neutron	0	1.00867	1.6744×10^{-27}	939.07

[a] amu = 1 atomic mass unit = 1.66×10^{-27} kg = 1/12 of the mass of ^{12}C.

[b] 1 atomic mass unit = 931 MeV.

Radioactive Decay

Radionuclides are unstable due to the unsuitable composition of neutrons and protons, or excess energy, and therefore, decay by emission of radiations such as α particles, β^- particles, β^+ particles, electron capture, and isomeric transition.

α decay: This decay occurs in heavy nuclei such as ^{235}U, ^{239}Pu, etc. For example,

$$^{235}_{92}U \rightarrow {}^{231}_{90}Th + \alpha \tag{1.1}$$

Alpha particles are a nucleus of helium atom having 2 protons and 2 neutrons in the nucleus with two orbital electrons stripped off from the K-shell. The α particles are emitted with discrete energy and have a very short range in matter, e.g., about 0.03 mm in human tissues.

β decay: β^- decay occurs in radionuclides that are neutron rich. In the process, a neutron in the nucleus is converted to a proton along with the emission of a β^- particle and an anti-neutrino, $\bar{\nu}$.

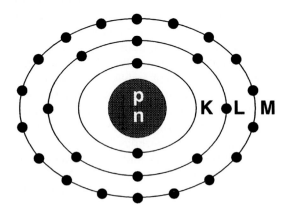

FIGURE 1-1. Schematic structure of a ^{28}Ni atom. The nucleus containing protons and neutrons is at the center. The K-shell has 2 electrons, the L-shell 8 electrons, and the M-shell 18 electrons.

$$n \rightarrow p + \beta^- + \bar{\nu} \tag{1.2}$$

For example,

$$^{131}_{53}I_{78} \rightarrow ^{131}_{54}Xe_{77} + \beta^- + \bar{\nu}$$

The energy difference between the two nuclides (i.e., between ^{131}I and ^{131}Xe in the above example) is called the decay energy or transition energy, which is shared between the β^- particle and the antineutrino $\bar{\nu}$. Therefore, β^- particles are emitted with a spectrum of energy with the transition energy as the maximum energy, and with an average energy equal to one-third of the maximum energy.

Positron (β⁺) decay: When a radionuclide is proton rich, it decays by the emission of a positron (β^+) along with a neutrino ν. In essence, a proton in the nucleus is converted to a neutron in the process.

$$p \rightarrow n + \beta^+ + \nu \tag{1.3}$$

Since a neutron is one electron mass heavier than a proton, the right-hand side of Eq. (1.3) is two electron mass more than the left-hand side, i.e., $2 \times 0.511\,MeV = 1.022\,MeV$ more on the right side. For conservation of energy, therefore, the radionuclide must have a transition energy of at least $1.022\,MeV$ to decay by β^+ emission. The energy beyond $1.022\,MeV$ is shared as kinetic energy by the β^+ particle and the neutrino.

Some examples of positron-emitting nuclides are:

$$^{18}_{9}F_9 \rightarrow ^{18}_{8}O_{10} + \beta^+ + \nu$$
$$^{82}_{37}Rb_{45} \rightarrow ^{82}_{36}Kr_{46} + \beta^+ + \nu$$

Positron emission tomography (PET) is based on the principle of coincidence detection of the two $511\,keV$ photons arising from positron emitters, which will be discussed in detail later.

Electron capture: When a radionuclide is proton rich, but has energy less than $1.022\,MeV$, then it decays by electron capture. In the process, an electron from the nearest shell, i.e., K-shell, is captured by a proton in the nucleus to produce a neutron.

$$p + e^- \rightarrow n + \nu \tag{1.4}$$

Note that when the transition energy is less than $1.022\,MeV$, the radionuclide definitely decays by electron capture. However, when the transition energy is more than $1.022\,MeV$, the radionuclide can decay by positron emission and/or electron capture. The greater the transition energy above $1.022\,MeV$, the more likely the radionuclide will decay by positron emission. Some examples of radionuclides decaying by electron capture are:

$$^{111}_{49}\text{In}+e^- \rightarrow \,^{111}_{48}\text{Cd}+v$$

$$^{67}_{31}\text{Ga}+e^- \rightarrow \,^{67}_{30}\text{Zn}+v$$

Isomeric transition: When a nucleus has excess energy above the ground state, it can exist in excited (energy) states, which are called the isomeric states. The lifetimes of these states normally are very short ($\sim 10^{-15}$ to 10^{-12} sec); however, in some cases, the lifetime can be longer in minutes to years. When an isomeric state has a longer lifetime, it is called a metastable state and is represented by "m." Thus, having an energy state of 140 keV above ^{99}Tc and decaying with a half-life of 6 hr, ^{99m}Tc is an isomer of ^{99}Tc.

$$^{99m}\text{Tc} \rightarrow \,^{99}\text{Tc}+\gamma$$

$$^{113m}\text{In} \rightarrow \,^{113}\text{In}+\gamma$$

A radionuclide may decay by α, β^-, β^+ emissions, or electron capture to different isomeric states of the product nucleus, if allowed by the rules of quantum physics. Naturally, these isomeric states decay to lower isomeric states and finally to the ground states of the product nucleus, and the energy differences appear as γ-ray photons.

As an alternative to γ-ray emission, the excitation energy may be transferred to an electron, preferably in the K-shell, which is then ejected with energy $E_\gamma - E_B$, where E_γ and E_B are the γ-ray energy and binding energy of the electron, respectively. (Figure 1-2) This process is called the internal conversion, and the ejected electron is called the conversion electron. The

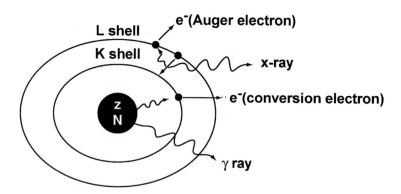

FIGURE 1-2. γ-ray emission and internal conversion process. In internal conversion process, the excitation energy of the nucleus is transferred to a K-shell electron, which is then ejected, and the K-shell vacancy is filled by an electron from the L-shell. The energy difference between the L-shell and K-shell appears as the characteristic K x-ray. The characteristic K x-ray energy may be transferred to an L-shell electron, which is then ejected in the Auger process.

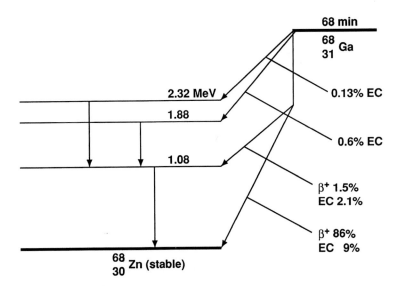

FIGURE 1-3. The decay scheme of ⁶⁸Ga. The 87.5% of positrons are annihilated to give rise to 175% of 511keV photons.

vacancy created in the *K*-shell is filled by the transition of an electron from an upper shell. The energy difference between the two shells appears as a characteristic *K* x-ray. Similarly, characteristic *L* x-ray, *M* x-ray, etc. can be emitted if the vacancy in the *L* or *M* shell is filled by electron transition from upper shells. Like *γ* rays, the characteristic x-ray energy can be emitted as photons or be transferred to an electron in a shell which is then ejected, if energetically possible. The latter is called the Auger process, and the ejected electron is called the Auger electron.

The decay of radionuclides is represented by a decay scheme, an example of which is given in Figure 1-3.

Radioactive Decay Equations

General Decay Equations

The atoms of a radioactive sample will decay randomly, and one cannot tell which atom will decay when. One can only talk about an average decay of the atoms in the sample. This decay rate is proportional to the number of radioactive atoms present. Mathematically,

$$-\frac{dN}{dt} = \lambda N \qquad (1.5)$$

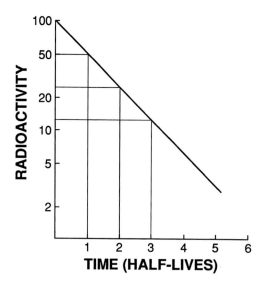

FIGURE 1-4. Plot of activity A_t against time on a semi-logarithmic graph indicating a straight line. The slope of the line is the decay constant λ of the radionuclide. The half-life $t_{1/2}$ is calculated from λ using Eq. (1. 8). Alternatively, the half-life is determined by reading an initial activity and half its value and their corresponding times. The difference in time between the two readings is the half-life.

where $-\dfrac{dN}{dt}$ is the rate of decay denoted by the term activity A, λ is the decay constant, and N is the number of atoms of the radionuclide present. Thus,

$$A = \lambda N \tag{1.6}$$

Integrating Eq. (1.5) gives the activity A_t at time t as

$$A_t = A_o e^{-\lambda t} \tag{1.7}$$

where A_o is the activity at time $t = 0$. The plot of A_t versus t on a semi-log scale is shown in Figure 1-4. If one knows activity A_o at a given time, the activity A_t at time t before or later can be calculated by Eq. (1.7).

Half-life ($t_{1/2}$): The half-life of a radionuclide is defined as the time required to reduce the initial activity to one-half. It is unique for every radionuclide and is related to the decay constant as follows:

$$\lambda = \frac{0.693}{t_{1/2}} \tag{1.8}$$

The half-life of a radionuclide is determined by measuring the radioactivity at different time intervals and plotting them on semi-logarithmic paper, as shown in Figure 1.4. An initial activity and half its value are read from the straight line, and the corresponding times are noted. The difference in time between the two readings gives the half-life of the radionuclide.

The mean life τ of a radionuclide is defined by

$$\tau = \frac{1}{\lambda} = \frac{t_{1/2}}{0.693} = 1.44 t_{1/2} \tag{1.9}$$

A radionuclide decays by 63% in one mean life.

Effective half-life: Each radionuclide decays with a definite half-life, called the physical half-life, which is denoted by T_P or $t_{1/2}$. When radiopharmaceuticals are administered to patients, analogous to physical decay, they are eliminated from the body by biological processes such as fecal excretion, urinary excretion, perspiration, etc. This elimination is characterized by a biological half-life (T_b) which is defined as the time taken to eliminate a half of the administered activity from the biological system. It is related to the decay constant λ_b by

$$\lambda_b = \frac{0.693}{T_b}$$

Thus, in a biological system, the loss of a radiopharmaceutical is related to λ_p and λ_b. The net effective rate of loss (λ_e) is characterized by

$$\lambda_e = \lambda_p + \lambda_b \tag{1.10}$$

Since $\lambda = 0.693/t_{1/2}$,

$$\frac{1}{T_e} = \frac{1}{T_p} + \frac{1}{T_b} \tag{1.11}$$

$$T_e = \frac{T_p \times T_b}{T_p + T_b} \tag{1.12}$$

The effective half-life is always less than the shorter of T_p or T_b. For a very long T_p and a short T_b, T_e is almost equal to T_b. Similarly, for a very long T_b and a short T_p, T_e is almost equal to T_p.

Successive Decay Equations

In a successive decay, a parent radionuclide p decays to a daughter nuclide d, and d in turn decays to another nuclide c, and we are interested in the decay rate of d over time. Thus,

$$p \rightarrow d \rightarrow c$$

Mathematically,

$$-\frac{dN_d}{dt} = \lambda_p N_p - \lambda_d N_d \tag{1.13}$$

On integration,

$$A_d = \frac{\lambda_d (A_p)_o}{\lambda_d - \lambda_p} \left[e^{-\lambda_p t} - e^{-\lambda_d t} \right] \tag{1.14}$$

If the parent half-life is greater than the daughter half-life (say a factor of 10 to 100), and also if the time of decay (t) is very long, then $e^{-\lambda_d t}$ is almost zero compared to $e^{-\lambda_p t}$. Then

$$(A_d)_t = \frac{\lambda_d}{\lambda_d - \lambda_p} (A_p)_t \tag{1.15}$$

Equation (1.15) represents a *transient equilibrium* between the parent *p* and daughter *d* radionuclides, which is achieved after several half-lives of the daughter. The graphical representation of this equilibrium is shown in Figure 1-5. It can be seen that after equilibrium, the daughter activity is greater than the parent activity and the daughter appears to decay follow-

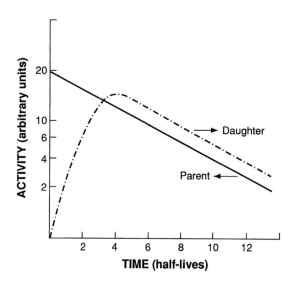

FIGURE 1-5. The transient equilibrium is illustrated in the plot of activity versus time on a semi-logarithmic graph. The daughter activity increases initially with time, reaches a maximum, then transient equilibrium, and finally appears to follow the half-life of the parent. Note that the daughter activity is higher than the parent activity in equilibrium.

ing the half-life of the parent. The principle of transient equilibrium is applied to many radionuclide generators such as the ^{99}Mo-^{99m}Tc generator.

If the parent half-life is much greater than the daughter half-life (by factors of hundreds or thousands), then λ_p is very negligible compared to λ_d. Then Eq. (1.15) becomes

$$(A_d)_t = (A_p)_t \tag{1.16}$$

This equation represents a *secular equilibrium* in which the daughter activity becomes equal to the parent activity, and the daughter decays with the half-life of the parent. The ^{82}Sr-^{82}Rb generator is an example of secular equilibrium.

Units of Radioactivity

$1\,Ci = 3.7 \times 10^{10}$ disintegration per sec (dps)
$1\,mCi = 3.7 \times 10^{7}\,dps$
$1\,\mu Ci = 3.7 \times 10^{4}\,dps$

Units of Radioactivity in System Internationale

1 Becquerel (Bq) $= 1\,dps$
$1\,kBq = 10^{3}\,dps = 2.7 \times 10^{-8}\,Ci$
$1\,MBq = 10^{6}\,dps = 2.7 \times 10^{-5}\,Ci$
$1\,GBq = 10^{9}\,dps = 2.7 \times 10^{-2}\,Ci$

Calculations

Problem 1.1

A dosage of ^{18}F-FDG has 20mCi at 10 a.m. Wednesday. Calculate the activity of the dosage at 7 a.m. and 2 p.m. that day. The half-life of ^{18}F is 110 minutes.

Answer:

$$\lambda \text{ for } {}^{18}\text{F} = \frac{0.693}{110} \text{ min}^{-1}$$

time from 7 a.m. to 10 a.m. $= 3\,hrs$
$= 180\,min$
time from 10 a.m. to 2 a.m. $= 4\,hrs$
$= 240\,min$

Activity of ^{18}F-FDG at 7 a.m. $= 20 \times e^{+\frac{0.693}{110} \times 180}$

$= 20 \times e^{+1.134}$

$= 62\,mCi\ (2.29\,GBq)$

Activity of ^{18}F-FDG at 2 p.m. $= 20 \times e^{-\frac{0.693 \times 240}{110}}$

$$= 20 \times e^{-1.512}$$
$$= 20 \times 0.22$$
$$= 4.4 \text{ mCi (163.1 MBq)}$$

Problem 1.2

A radioactive sample decays 40% per hour. What is the half-life of the radionuclide?

Answer:

$$\lambda = 0.4\text{hr}^{-1} = \frac{0.693}{t_{1/2}}$$

$$t_{1/2} = \frac{0.693}{0.4}$$
$$= 1.73\text{hr}$$

Interaction of Radiation with Matter

Radiations are either particulate type, such as α particle, β particle, etc. or nonparticulate type, such as electromagnetic radiation (e.g γ rays, infrared rays, x-rays, etc.), and both kinds are ionizing radiations. The mode of inter-action of these two types of radiations with matter is different.

Interaction of Charged Particles with Matter

The energetic charged particles such as α particles and β particles, while passing through matter, lose their energy by interacting with the orbital electrons of the atoms in the matter. In these processes, the atoms are ionized in which the electron in the encounter is ejected, or are excited in which the electron is raised to a higher energy state. In both excitation and ionization processes, chemical bonds in the molecules of the matter may be ruptured, forming a variety of chemical entities.

The lighter charged particles (e.g., β particles) move in a zigzag path in the matter, whereas the heavier particles (e.g., α particles) move in a straight path, because of the heavy mass and charge. The straight line path traversed by the charged particles is called the range R. The range of a charged particle depends on the energy, charge and mass of the particle as well as the density of the matter it passes through. It increases with increas-ing charge and energy, while it decreases with increasing mass of the parti-cle and increasing density of the matter. The range of positrons and other properties of common positron-emitters are given in Table 1.2.

TABLE 1.2. Properties of common positron emitters.

Radionuclide range	Half-life	$E_{\beta,max}^+$ (MeV)	Max. β^+ range (mm) in water	Average β^+ (mm) in water
^{11}C	20.4 min	0.97	3.8	0.85
^{13}N	10 min	1.20	5.0	1.15
^{15}O	2 min	1.74	8.0	1.80
^{18}F	110 min	0.64	2.2	0.46
^{68}Ga	68 min	1.90	9.0	2.15
^{82}Rb	75 sec	3.35	15.5	4.10

Adapted by the permission of the Society of Nuclear Medicine from: Brown TF and Yasillo NJ. Radiation safety considerations for PET centers. J Nucl Med Technol 1997;25:98.

A unique situation of the passage of positrons through an absorber is that as a positron loses its energy by interaction with electrons of the absorber atoms and comes to almost rest, it combines with an electron of an absorber atom. At this instant, both particles (β^+ and e^-) are annihilated to produce two photons of 511 keV, which are emitted in opposite directions (~180°) (Figure 1-6). This process is called the *annihilation* process. Detection of the two opposite 511 keV photons in coincidence by two detectors is the basis of positron emission tomography (PET).

BETA PLUS DECAY

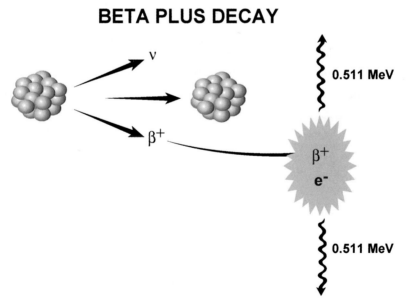

FIGURE 1-6. A schematic illustration of the annihilation of a positron and an electron in the medium. Two 511 keV photons are produced and emitted in opposite directions (180°). (Reprinted with the permission of the Cleveland Clinic Foundation.)

An important parameter related to the interaction of radiations with matter is linear energy transfer (LET). It is the energy deposited by a radiation per unit length of the path in the absorber and is normally given in units of kiloelectron volt per micrometer (*keV/μm*). The LET varies with the energy, charge and mass of the particle. The γ radiations and β^- particles interact with matter depositing relatively less amount of energy per unit length and so have low LET. On the other hand, α particles, protons, etc. deposit more energy per unit length because of their greater mass and charge, and so have higher LET.

Interaction of γ Radiation With Matter

In the spectrum of electromagnetic radiations, γ radiations are high-frequency radiations and interact with matter by three mechanisms: photoelectric, Compton, and pair production.

Photoelectric process: In this process, a γ radiation, while passing through an absorber, transfers its entire energy primarily to an inner shell electron (e.g. the K-shell) of an absorber atom and ejects the electron (Figure 1-7). The ejected electron will have the kinetic energy equal to $E_\gamma - E_B$, where E_γ is the γ-ray energy and E_B is the binding energy of the electron in the shell. The probability of this process decreases with increasing energy of the γ ray, but increases with increasing atomic number of the absorber. It is roughly given by Z^5/E_γ^3. The vacancy in the shell is filled in by the transition of an electron from the upper shell, which is followed by emission of the energy difference between the two shells as characteristic x-rays, or by the Auger process described in the internal conversion process.

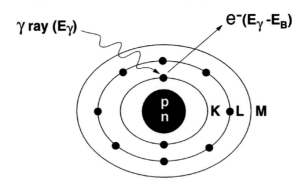

Photoelectric Process

FIGURE 1-7. An illustration of photoelectric effect, where a γ ray transfers all its energy E_γ to a K-shell electron, and the electron is ejected with $E_\gamma - E_B$, where E_B is the binding energy of the electron in the K-shell. The characteristic K x-ray emission or the Auger process can follow, as described in Figure 1-2.

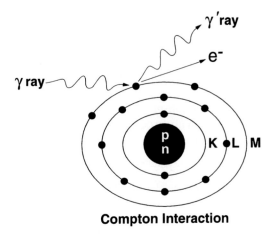

Compton Interaction

FIGURE 1-8. The Compton scattering process in which a γ ray transfers only a part of its energy to an electron in a shell and is itself scattered with reduced energy. The electron is ejected from the shell with energy, $E'_\gamma - E_B$, where E'_γ is the partial energy transferred by the γ ray and E_B is the binding energy of the electron in the shell. The remaining γ-ray energy appears as a scattered photon.

Compton Scattering Process: In a Compton scattering process, a γ radiation with somewhat higher energy interacts with an outer shell electron of the absorber atom transferring only part of its energy to the electron and ejecting it (Figure 1-8). The ejected electron is called the Compton electron and carries a part of the γ-ray energy minus its binding energy in the shell, i.e., $E'_\gamma - E_B$, where E'_γ is the partial energy of the original γ ray. The remaining energy of the γ ray will appear as a scattered photon. Thus, in Compton scattering, a scattered photon and a Compton electron are produced. The scattered photon may again encounter a photoelectric process or another Compton scattering process, or leave the absorber without interaction. As the energy of the γ radiation increases, the photoelectric process decreases and the Compton scattering process increases, but the latter also decreases with photon energy above 1.0 MeV or so. The probability of Compton scattering is independent of the atomic number Z of the absorber.

Pair Production: When the γ-ray energy is higher than 1.022 MeV, the photon interacts with the nucleus of an absorber atom during its passage through it and produces a positron and an electron. This is called pair production. The excess energy beyond 1.022 MeV is shared as kinetic energy between the two particles. The probability of pair production increases with increasing photon energy above 1.022 MeV. The positron produced will undergo annihilation in the absorber as described earlier.

Attenuation of γ Radiations

When γ radiations pass through the absorber medium, they undergo one or a combination of the above three processes (photoelectric, Compton, and pair production) depending on their energy, or they are transmitted out of the absorber without any interaction. The combined effect of the 3 processes is called the *attenuation* of the γ radiations (Figure 1-9). For a γ radiation passing through an absorber, the linear attenuation coefficient (μ_t) of the γ radiation is given by

$$\mu_l = \tau + \sigma + \kappa \tag{1.17}$$

where τ is the photoelectric coefficient, σ is the Compton coefficient and κ is the pair production coefficient (Figure 1-10). The linear attenuation coefficient of a radiation in an absorber has the unit of cm^{-1}, and normally decreases with energy and increases with the atomic number and density of the absorber. If a photon beam I_o passes through an absorber of thickness x, then the transmitted beam (I_x) is given by

$$I_x = I_o e^{-\mu_l x} \tag{1.18}$$

The attenuation of a photon beam in human tissues during imaging is a critical factor to consider in both single photon emission computed tomography (SPECT) or PET, which will be discussed later.

An important quantity in the discussion of photon interaction with matter is the half-value layer (HVL), which is defined as the thickness of the absorber that attenuates an initial photon beam intensity to one-half. The HVL increases with higher energy of the photon and decreases with increasing atomic number of the absorber. Lead is a high atomic number

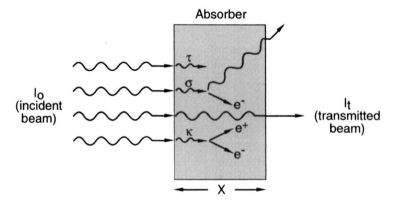

FIGURE 1-9. Illustration of attenuation of a photon beam (I_o) in an absorber of thickness x. Attenuation comprises photoelectric effect (τ), Compton scattering (σ) and pair production (κ). Photons passing through the absorber without interaction constitute the transmitted beam (I_t).

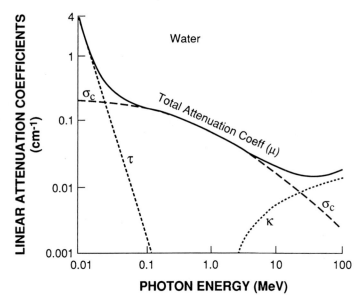

FIGURE 1-10. Linear attenuation coefficient of γ rays of different energies in water (equivalent to body tissue). The relative contributions of photoelectric, Compton scattering and pair production processes are illustrated.

inexpensive metal that has very high absorbing power for γ radiations providing low HVL values and that is why it is commonly used for radiation protection. The HVL is related to the linear attenuation coefficient as follows:

$$\mu_\ell = \frac{0.693}{HVL} \tag{1.19}$$

The HVL for 511 keV photons in some absorbers are given in Table 1.3.

Along the same line, the tenth-value layer (TVL) is defined by the thickness of the absorber that reduces the initial intensity of the photons by a factor of 10. It is given by

$$TVL = \frac{-\ln(0.1)}{\mu_\ell}$$
$$= \frac{2.30}{\mu_\ell}$$
$$= 3.32\, HVL \tag{1.20}$$

Another quantity called the mass attenuation coefficient (μ_g) is given by the linear attenuation coefficient (μ_ℓ) divided by the density (ρ) of the absorber and is given in units of cm^2/g or cm^2/mg.

TABLE 1.3. Half-value layers of 511 keV photons in different absorber materials.

Absorber material	HVL (mm) (narrow beam)	HVL (mm)* (broad beam)
Lead	4.1	5.5
Tungsten	—	3.2
Iron	—	16.0
Concrete	33.2	8.7
Tissue	7.1	—

* Adapted from Townson JEC. Radiation dosimetry and protection in PET. In: Valk PE, Bailey DL, Townsend DW, Maisey MN, eds. *Positron Emission Tomography*. New York: Springer-Verlag; 2003.

Thus,

$$\mu_g = \frac{\mu_e}{\rho} \qquad (1.21)$$

Questions

1. The total number of nucleons in an atom is designated by (A) N; (B) Z; (C) M; (D) A.
2. Isotopes contain the same number of _____.
3. Isobars contain the same number of _____.
4. ^{99m}Tc and ^{99}Tc are two _____.
5. Isomeric transition is an alternative to gamma ray emission. True _____; False _____.
6. Gamma ray emission is an alternative to internal conversion. True _____; False _____.
7. Describe the Auger process in radioactive decay.
8. Name two nuclear decay processes in which characteristic x-rays are possibly emitted.
9. What types of radionuclides are designated as metastable isomers with symbol "m" in the mass number?
10. Why is a neutrino needed in the positron decay? In what decay is an antineutrino emitted?
11. In a β^- decay, the transition energy is 400 keV. The β^- particle is emitted with 315 keV. What is the energy of the antineutrino?
12. Describe the annihilation process.
13. Explain why two photons of 511 keV are emitted in positron annihilation.
14. If a K-shell electron whose binding energy is 25 keV is emitted as a result of internal conversion of a 135 keV photon, what is the energy of the ejected electron?

15. What types of radionuclides would decay by β^- and β^+ emission and electron capture?

16. How long will it take for the decay of three-quarters of a ^{18}F-FDG ($t_{1/2} = 110$min) sample?

17. What are the conditions for transient equilibrium and secular equilibrium in radioactive decay?

18. If the activity of ^{18}F-FDG is 25mCi at 10 a.m. Wednesday, what is the activity at 2:30 p.m. the same day ($t_{1/2}$ of ^{18}F = 110min)?

19. ^{18}F-FDG dosages are shipped from a vendor 3 hours away from the customer. What initial amount should be sent in order to have a 10mCi dosage for the customer?

20. A radioactive sample initially gives 9500cpm and 3 hours later 2500 cpm. Calculate the half-life of the radionuclides.

21. ^{18}F-FDG has a biological half-life of 10 hours in humans and a physical half-life of 110 minutes. What is the effective $t_{1/2}$ of the radiopharmaceutical?

22. Define linear energy transfer (LET) and range (R) of charged particles.

23. The range of a charged particulate radiation in matter increases:
    (a) as the mass increases True _____; False _____
    (b) as the charge increases True _____; False _____
    (c) as the energy decreases True _____; False _____

24. Describe photoelectric and Compton scattering processes.

25. The photoelectric interaction of a γ ray increases with:
    (a) energy True _____; False _____
    (b) atomic number of the absorber True _____; False _____

26. A 350keV γ ray interacts with a K-shell electron by the photoelectric interaction. If the binding energy of the K-shell electron is 25keV, what is the kinetic energy of the photoelectron?

27. Does Compton scattering depend on the atomic number of the absorber?

28. (a) Describe attenuation of a photon beam through an absorber.
    (b) Does it depend on density and atomic number of the absorber?
    (c) Define linear attenuation coefficient and half-value layer of a γ ray in an absorber.

29. If 1mCi of a radionuclide is adequately shielded by 6HVLs of lead, how many HVLs would be needed to have equal shielding for (a) 5mCi and (b) 8mCi of the radionuclide?

30. How many HVLs are approximately equivalent to three tenth-value layers?

31. If 15% of the 511keV photons of ^{18}F are transmitted after passing through a lead brick of 7cm thickness, calculate the HVL of the 511keV photon in lead.

References and Suggested Reading

1. Bushberg JT, Seibert JA, Leidholdt, EM Sr, Boone JM. *The Essential Physics of Medical Imaging*. 2nd ed. Philadelphia: Lippincott, Williams & Wilkins; 2002.
2. Cherry SR, Sorenson JA, Phelps ME. *Physics in Nuclear Medicine*. 3rd ed. Philadelphia: W.B. Saunders; 2003.
3. Friedlander G, Kennedy JW, Miller JM. *Nuclear and Radiochemistry*. 3rd ed. New York: Wiley; 1981.
4. Saha GB. *Physics and Radiobiology of Nuclear Medicine*. 2nd ed. New York: Springer-Verlag; 2001.

2
PET Scanning Systems

Background

The detection and measurement of radiation is based on the interaction of radiations with matter, as discussed in the last chapter. In gases, ionizing radiations, particulate or electromagnetic, interact with gas molecules to produce positive and negative ions, which are then collected as current or counts by the application of a voltage. The amount of ionization is proportional to the amount of energy deposited by the radiation. At low voltages, the ionization is measured as current that is proportional to the amount of radiation. Dose calibrators, pocket dosimeters, and ionization chambers operate on this principle at low voltages (~150 V). At high voltages (~900 V), ions are multiplied in an avalanche of interactions producing a pulse that is independent of the energy and type of radiation. Each event of interaction is detected as a count, and this principle is applied in Geiger-Müller (GM) counters, which are used as radiation survey meters.

Liquid scintillation detectors operate on the principle of interaction of radiations with a special type of scintillating liquid that emits light upon interaction with radiation. The light is then processed in the same manner as in the case of a solid detector, as discussed below.

Both gas and liquid scintillation detectors have low detection efficiency and, therefore, are not used in PET technology. Interaction of radiations with solid scintillation detectors is the basis of radiation detection in PET technology. These solid detectors have the unique property of emitting scintillation or flashes of light after absorbing γ or x-ray radiations. The light photons are converted to an electrical pulse or signal by a photomultiplier (PM) tube. The pulse is further amplified by a linear amplifier, sorted by a pulse height analyzer (PHA), and then registered as a count. Different types of radiations are detected by different types of detectors. For example, γ rays or x-rays are detected by sodium iodide crystal containing a trace amount of thallium, NaI(Tl), whereas organic scintillation detectors such as anthracene and plastic fluor are used for β^- particle detection. PET is based on the detection of two 511 keV photons in coincidence at 180°. These photons are produced by the annihilation process, in which a positron emitted by a positron-emitting radionuclide combines with an electron in the medium and is annihilated. Solid scintillation detectors of different materials have been investigated to detect 511 keV photons. The following is a brief description of the properties and uses of solid detectors in PET imaging.

Solid Scintillation Detectors in PET

Although many solid scintillation detectors have been investigated, only a few have been widely used in PET technology. The characteristics of different detectors that have application in PET technology are listed in Table 2.1. The choice of a detector is based on several characteristics, namely:

1. Stopping power of the detector for 511 keV photons,
2. Scintillation decay time.
3. Light output per keV of photon energy,
4. Energy resolution of the detector.

The stopping power of the detector determines the mean distance the photon travels until it stops after complete deposition of its energy, and depends on the density and effective atomic number (Z_{eff}) of the detector material. The scintillation decay time arises when a γ ray interacts with an atom of the detector material, and the atom is excited to a higher energy level, which later decays to the ground state, emitting visible light. This time of decay is called the scintillation decay time given in nanoseconds (ns) and varies with the material of the detector. The shorter the decay time, the higher the efficiency of the detector at high count rates. A high-light-output

TABLE 2.1. Physical properties of common PET scintillator detectors.

Property	NaI (Tl)	BGO	LSO	YSO	GSO	BaF$_2$
Effective Z	50	74	66	34	59	52
Density (gm/cm³)	3.7	7.1	7.4	4.5	6.7	4.9
Scintillation decay time (ns)	230	300	40	70	60	0.6
Photon yield per keV	38	6	29	46	10	2
Relative light output	100	15	75	118	25	5
Linear attenuation coefficient, μ(cm⁻¹)	0.35	0.96	0.87	0.39	0.70	0.44
Energy resolution (% at 511 keV)	6.6	20	10	12.5	8.5	11.4

BGO: Bismuth Germanate, $Bi_4Ge_3O_{12}$.
LSO: Lutetium oxyorthosilicate doped with cerium (Ce), Lu_2SiO_5:Ce.
YSO: Yttrium oxyorthosilicate doped with Ce, Y_2SiO_5:Ce.
GSO: Gadolinium oxyorthosilicate doped with Ce, Gd_2SiO_5:Ce.
BaF$_2$: Barium fluoride.

detector produces a well-defined pulse resulting in better energy resolution. The intrinsic energy resolution is affected by inhomogeneities in the crystal structure of the detector and random variations in the production of light in it. The energy resolutions at 511 keV in different detectors vary from 6% to 20% (Table 2.1), for routine integration time of pulse formation, which runs around a few microseconds. However, in PET imaging, the integration time is a few hundred nanoseconds in order to exclude random coincidences, and the number of photoelectrons collected for a pulse is small, thus degrading the energy resolution. Consequently, the detectors in PET scanners have relatively poorer energy resolution (10% to 25%), and these values are given in Table 2.2 for scanners from different manufacturers.

The detection efficiency of a detector is another important property in PET technology. Since it is desirable to have shorter scan times and low tracer activity for administration, the detector must detect as many of the emitted photons as possible. The 511 keV photons interact with detector material by either photoelectric absorption or Compton scattering, as discussed in Chapter 1. Thus, the photons are attenuated (absorbed and scattered) by these two processes in the detector, and the fraction of incident γ rays that are attenuated is determined by the linear attenuation coefficient (μ) given in Chapter 1 and gives the detection efficiency. At 511 keV, $\mu = 0.96\,\text{cm}^{-1}$ for bismuth germanate (BGO), $0.87\,\text{cm}^{-1}$ for lutetium oxyorthosilicate (LSO), and $0.35\,\text{cm}^{-1}$ for NaI(Tl) (Melcher, 2000). Consequently, to have similar detection efficiency, NaI(Tl) detectors must be more than twice as thick as BGO and LSO detectors.

For γ-ray detection, NaI(Tl) detectors are most commonly used, as they provide good light output (30 to 40 light photons per keV of γ-ray energy) and energy resolution. They are most widely used in most gamma cameras for planar or single photon emission computed tomography (SPECT) imaging in nuclear medicine. The NaI(Tl) crystal is hygroscopic and, therefore, hermetically sealed with aluminum foil. It is fragile and needs careful handling. Its major drawback is its poor stopping power, i.e., low density and low linear attenuation coefficient for 511 keV. For this reason, though used in earlier PET systems, it has not received much appreciation for application in PET technology.

BGO detectors are used in most of the PET systems because of its highest stopping power (higher density and linear attenuation coefficient). However, it suffers from its longer scintillation decay time (~300 ns) and poor light output. The longer decay time increases the dead time of the detector and limits the count rate that can be detected by the system. The low light output results in poor energy resolution, which is proportional to the square root of the number of scintillation photons and is typically 20% for 511 keV photons.

The three characteristics of cerium-doped LSO, namely high light output, high stopping power (high density and large linear attenuation coefficient),

TABLE 2.2. Features of Different PET Scanners[§].

Feature	ADVANCE/ADVANCE Nxi (General Electric)	ECAT ACCEL (CTI-Siemens)	ECAT EXACT HR+ (CTI-Siemens)	ECAT EXACT (CTI-Siemens)	ECAT ART (CTI-Siemens)	C-PET (Philips-ADAC)	ALLEGRO (Philips-ADAC)
Number of rings	18	24	32	24	24	N/A	29
Ring diameter (mm)	927	824	824	824	824	900	860
Patient port (mm)	590	562	562	562	600	560	565
Crystals number	12,096	9,216	18,432	9,216	4,224	6	17,864
Crystal material	BGO	LSO	BGO	BGO	BGO	Curved NaI(Tl)[†]	GSO[*]
Crystal size (mm)	$4.0 \times 8.1 \times 30$	$6.45 \times 6.45 \times 25$	$4.05 \times 4.39 \times 30$	$6.29 \times 6.29 \times 20$	$6.29 \times 6.29 \times 20$	$500 \times 300 \times 25.4$	$4 \times 6 \times 20$
PMTs number	672 (dual)	576	1,152	576	264	288	420
Crystals/block	36	64	64	64	64	N/A	No blocks
Energy window width (keV)	300–650	350–650	350–650	350–650	350–650	435–665	435–560
Energy resolution (FWHM)	~25%	~25%	~25%	~25%	~25%	10%	15%
Coincidence window (ns)	12.5	6	12	12	12	8	8
Acquisition mode	2D/3D	2D/3D	2D/3D	2D/3D	3D	Full 3D	Full 3D
Transaxial FOV (mm)	550	585	585	583	600	576[‡]	576
Axial FOV (mm)	152	162	155	162	162	256	180
Number of image planes	35	47	63	47	47	64/128	90
Slice thickness (mm)	4.25	3.375	2.46	3.375	3.375	2	2
Septa material	Tungsten	Lead	Lead	Lead	N/A	N/A	N/A
Septa dimensions (mm)	1×117	1×65	0.5×65	1×65	N/A	N/A	N/A
Whole body scan length (cm)	170	195	195	195	195	168	198

[§] Reprinted by permission of the Society of Nuclear Medicine from: Tarantola et al. PET instrumentation and reconstruction algorithms in whole-body applications. *J Nucl Med.* 2003;44:756–769.
[*] PIXELAR.
[†] CCT.
[‡] 256 for brain imaging.
N/A = not applicable.

and short scintillation decay time (40ns) have made it an ideal detector for PET systems. However, owing to its intrinsic property, its energy resolution is poor despite its high light output. A disadvantage of this detector is that it contains a naturally occurring radioisotope of its own, [176]Lu, with an abundance of 2.6% and a half-life of 3.8×10^8 years. This radionuclide decays by emission of β^- rays and x-rays of 88 to 400keV. However, the activity level is too low to be concerned regarding radiation exposure from [176]Lu, and it does not pose any problem in PET imaging because its photon energy is lower than 511keV.

The overall characteristics of cerium-doped gadolinium oxyorthosilicate (GSO) detectors are quite good for application in PET technology. Even though it has lower light output and stopping power than the LSO detector, its better energy resolution has prompted some commercial manufacturers to use this detector in PET technology. Fabrication of GSO detectors requires great care, because the crystals are fragile. GSO detectors collect data faster than other materials and hence are often called "fast crystal." These detectors can be cut into smaller crystals resulting in improved spatial resolution of the system.

Barium fluoride (BaF_2) has the shortest decay time of 0.6ns and is primarily used in time-of-flight scanners that are rarely used clinically nowadays, because of various technical difficulties.

Cerium-doped yittrium oxyorthosilicate (YSO) is a new type of detector, but no commercial manufacturer has yet used it in PET technology.

Some promising detectors such as cerium-doped lutetium iodide and cerium-doped lanthanum bromide are in the development stage. Also, to increase the spatial resolution in tomographic imaging, several scintillation crystals with different decay constants are coupled in layers to form a single dual-layered detector. GSO and BGO detectors and NaI(Tl) and LSO detectors have been coupled in this manner for high-resolution scanners. The latter dual detector can be used for either SPECT or PET scanning by switching between the two detectors.

Photomultiplier Tube

As discussed briefly earlier, a photomultiplier (PM) tube is needed to convert the light photons produced in the detector as a result of γ-ray interaction to an electrical pulse. The PM tube is a vacuum glass tube containing a photocathode at one end, 10 dynodes in the middle, and an anode at the other end, as shown in Figure 2-1. The photocathode is usually an alloy of cesium and antimony that releases electrons after absorption of light photons. The PM tube is fixed on to the detector by optical grease or optical light pipes.

A high voltage of ~1000 volts is applied between the photocathode and the anode, with about 100-volt increments between the dynodes. When light photons from the detector strike the photocathode of the PM tube, elec-

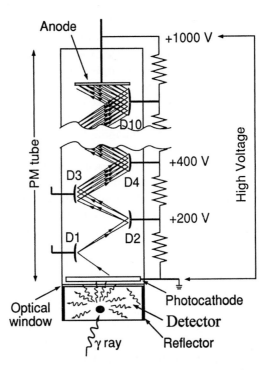

FIGURE 2-1. A photomultiplier tube showing the photocathode at one end, several dynodes inside, and an anode at the other end.

trons are emitted, which are accelerated toward the next closest dynode by the voltage difference between the dynodes. Approximately 1 to 3 electrons are emitted per 7 to 10 light photons. Each of these electrons is again accelerated toward the next dynode and then more electrons are emitted. The process of multiplication continues until the last dynode is reached and a pulse of electrons is produced, which is then attracted toward the anode. The pulse is then delivered to the preamplifier. Next, it is amplified by an amplifier to a detectable pulse, which is then analyzed for its size by the pulse height analyzer, and finally delivered to a recorder or computer for storage or to a monitor for display.

Pulse Height Analyzer

A pulse height analyzer (PHA) is a device that sorts out photons of different energies arising from either the individual photons of the same or different radionuclides, or from the scattered photons. Functionally, a PHA is a discriminator with a lower level and an upper level setting or with a baseline and a window above the baseline. In either setting, photons of selected energy only are accepted and others are rejected. This type of pulse sorting is essential in nuclear medicine imaging to count mainly unscattered photons that come out of the organ of interest for image formation. The narrower the window of the PHA, the more accurate is the energy discrimination of photons from the sample, but the detection efficiency is reduced. In the case of PET systems, the window of the PHA is centered around 511 keV, with a width of 350 keV to 650 keV.

Arrangement of Detectors

In the earlier designs of PET cameras, each detector (normally BGO) is glued to a single PM tube, and a large array of such detectors are arranged in multiple circular rings around the object of imaging. The axial field of view is defined by the width of the array of the rings, and the number of detectors per ring varies with the manufacturers. The total number of detectors ranges in the thousands, depending on the manufacturer. The larger the number of detectors and hence the more PM tubes per ring, the better the spatial resolution of the system. Although such systems provide good resolution, the cost of using many PM tubes is high, and packaging of a large number of detectors with PM tubes becomes impractical.

In modern PET scanners, the *block detector* has been designed and used, in which small detectors, created by partially cutting a large block of detector material, are utilized and the number of PM tubes is reduced. A schematic block detector is shown in Figure 2-2. Typically, each block detector is about 3 cm deep and grooved into an array of 6×8, 7×8, or 8×8 elements by making partial cuts through the crystal with a saw. The cuts are made at varying depths, with the deepest cut at the edge of the block. The

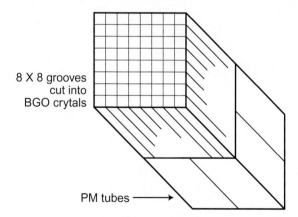

FIGURE 2-2. A schematic block detector is segmented into 8×8 elements, and 4PM tubes are coupled to the block for pulse formation. (Reprinted with the permission of the Cleveland Clinic Foundation.)

grooves between the elements are filled with an opaque reflective material that prevents optical spillover between elements but facilitates sharing of light among the PM tubes. The width of the detector elements determines the spatial resolution of the imaging device and is normally 3 to 5 mm in modern PET scanners. The entire block detector is attached to several PM tubes (normally 4 PM tubes) in the same fashion as in scintillation cameras. BGO block detectors can use up to 16 detector elements per PM tube, whereas LSO block detectors use up to 144 detector elements because of higher intensity of scintillation emission. A typical commercial block detector is shown in Figure 2-3. A PET scanner can contain many block detectors, the number of which varies with the manufacturer. These detectors are arranged in arrays in full rings or partial rings in different configurations discussed later. The number of rings varies from 18 to 32 depending on the manufacturer. The block detector design has the advantage of reduced dead time compared to those of the scintillation cameras because of the restricted light spread in the former.

A modification of the basic block detector has been made such that each PM tube straddles over four quadrants of four different blocks (Figure 2-4). The technique of quadrant sharing permits the use of larger PM tubes and reduces the total number of PM tubes used in the PET

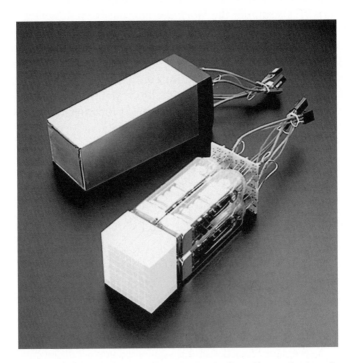

FIGURE 2-3. A typical commercial block detector (8 × 8) attached to four square PM tubes (bottom) and a packaged module (top), developed and manufactured by CPS Innovations. (Courtesy of CPS Innovations, Knoxville, TN, USA.)

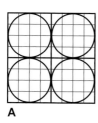

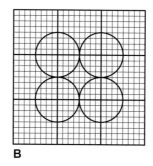

FIGURE 2-4. Block detector illustrating the quadrant sharing of PM tubes. (A) PM tubes assigned in 4 quadrants separately. (B) Each PM tube shares 4 quadrants of 4 block detectors and improves the spatial resolution. (Reprinted with the permission of the Cleveland Clinic Foundation.)

scanner. This design improves the spatial resolution relative to the basic design, but has the disadvantage of increasing the dead time.

In a PET scanner, each detector element is connected by a coincidence circuit with a time window to a set of opposite detector elements (both in plane and axial). Typically, the time window is set at 6ns to 20ns depending on the type of detector. If there are N detector elements in a ring, typically each detector is in coincidence with $N/2$ detector elements on the opposite side, and, therefore, $N/2$ "fan-beam" projections are available for each detector element (Figure 2-5). Note that less than $N/2$ detectors can be connected in coincidence. These fan-beam projections form for each

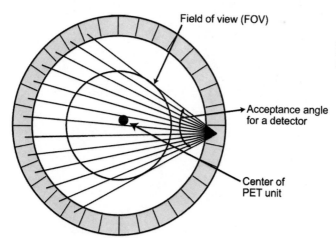

FIGURE 2-5. The transverse field of view determined by the acceptance angles of individual detectors in a PET scanner. Each detector is connected in coincidence with as many as half the total number of detectors in a ring and the data for each detector are acquired in a "fan beam" projection. All possible fan beam acquisitions are made for all detectors, which define the FOV as shown in the figure. (Reprinted with the permission of the Cleveland Clinic Foundation.)

detector an angle of acceptance in the transaxial plane, and these angles of acceptance for all detectors in the ring form the transaxial field of view (FOV). The larger the number of detectors (up to $N/2$) in multicoincidence with each detector, the larger the angle of acceptance and hence the larger transaxial FOV for the PET system.

PET Scanners

Dedicated PET scanners typically are designed with detectors (block detectors) arranged in an array of full or partial rings with a diameter of 80 to 90cm. The full ring geometry is realized in a circular or hexagonal form with either the use of block detectors (CTI or Siemens: ECAT EXACT HR$^+$ or GE ADVANCE) or the use of 6 curved detectors (NaI(Tl) has been used only in C-PET: Phillips-ADAC Medical). Another arrangement is Pixelar module, which is a curved matrix made of 628 (22×29 rings) GSO detectors coupled to 15PM tubes, and 28 such modules are used to make the ring (ALLEGRO: Phillips-ADAC Medical). Other systems include partial rings of two opposite curved matrices made of 33 (8×8) BGO detectors (11 tangentially and 3 axially) with a reciprocal 15° angular shift that increases the transverse field of view (FOV) during detector rotation (ECAT EXACT HR$^+$, CTI, Inc.). The configurations of detectors in some PET systems are

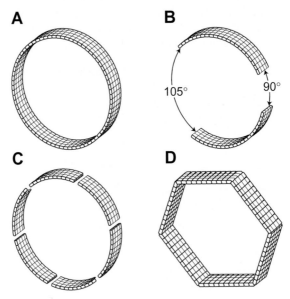

FIGURE 2-6. Different configurations of PET scanners. (A) A circular full-ring scanner. (B) A partial ring scanner with a 15° angular shift between two blocks of detectors. (C) Continuous detectors using curve plates of NaI(Tl). (D) Hexagonal array of quadrant-sharing panel detectors. (Reprinted with the permission of the Cleveland Clinic Foundation.)

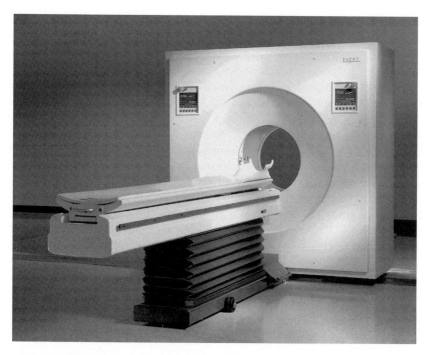

FigURE 2-7. A dedicated PET scanner developed and manufactured by CPS Innovations. (Courtesy of CPS Innovations, Knoxville, TN, USA.)

illustrated in Figure 2-6. Since PET scanners are axially fixed, whole-body scanners are equipped with a computer-controlled moving bed so that the patient can be positioned at different positions along the axial field for whole-body scanning. The whole body scan length varies from 170 cm to 198 cm depending on the manufacturer. Different PET scanners and their characteristics are listed in Table 2.2. A dedicated clinical PET scanner is shown in Figure 2.7.

Hybrid Scintillation Cameras

Conventional scintillation cameras using NaI(Tl) detectors are available in dual-head and triple-head designs to perform planar and single photon emission computed tomography (SPECT) imaging. To utilize them as PET systems, the heads of these cameras are connected with a coincidence circuitry. The coincidence time window is typically set at ~12ns for dual-head and ~10ns for triple-head cameras. Data are acquired by rotating the heads without the collimator around the subject. These units are capable of switching between PET and SPECT modes, of course, using the collimator in the latter mode. These hybrid systems are very attractive to the community hospitals because of the relatively low cost, while providing the scope for PET imaging.

A disadvantage of the hybrid systems is that they have low sensitivity due to low detection efficiency of NaI(Tl) crystal for 511 keV photons, which results in a longer acquisition time. To improve the sensitivity, thicker detectors of sizes 1.6 cm to 2.5 cm have been used in some cameras, but even then, coincidence photopeak efficiency is only 3% to 4%. This increase in crystal thickness, however, compromises the spatial resolution of the system in SPECT mode. Fast electronics and pulse shaping are implemented in modern systems to improve the sensitivity. Also, there is a significant camera dead time and pulse pile-ups due to relatively increased single count rates in the absence of a collimator in PET mode. A newly developed detector signal processing algorithm, called the high-yield pile-up event-recovery (HYPER), removes most pile-ups and thus gives higher counts. Low coincidence count rates due to low detection efficiency of NaI(Tl) detectors for 511 keV photons cause higher background noise that results in low contrast in the reconstructed image with hybrid systems, compared to dedicated PET scanners. The overall spatial resolution of the dual-head coincidence cameras is poorer than that of the PET scanners.

PET/CT Scanners

In the interpretation of nuclear medicine studies, physicians always prefer to have a comparison between high-resolution CT or MR images and low-resolution PET or SPECT images of a patient for precise localization of lesions. It is very useful to compare the images before and after therapy to assess the effectiveness of treatment. To this end, efforts are made to co-register two sets of digital images. In co-registration, the matrix size, voxel intensity, and the rotation are adjusted to establish a one-to-one spatial correspondence between the two images. This process is called the alignment of images. Several techniques are employed in alignment of images of different modalities, among which the following three are common: In the manual method, the contour of the two sets of images are traced and then the images are aligned; second, in the landmark technique, an external point marker that can be seen on both images is attached to the patient, or an internal marker such as a structure in an organ that is common to both images is chosen; third, in the fully automated method, surfaces or boundaries between organs are chosen by algorithms to define the images for alignment. This technique is useful for rigid body organs such as the brain, whereas it is likely to cause noises and hence errors in registration of the nonrigid, moving organs, such as the heart, abdomen, etc. Another important method of image alignment based on voxel intensities of the two images uses the difference in intensities or the standard deviations of the ratios of image intensities (voxel-by-voxel basis) for proper alignment of the two images. After alignment, the source image or each discrete point in the source image is transformed to the coordinate system of the target image (e.g., CT images transformed to PET images). This is done on a voxel-by-voxel basis. In all cases, algorithms have been developed and employed to achieve co-registration of images of different modalities. Most software is vendor-neutral and supports fusion of any combination of functional and anatomical images of different modalities. Some common software are: Siemens Medical Solutions' Syngo, Philips Medical's Syntegra, MIMvista's MIM, Mirada Solutions' Fusion 7D and Hermes Medical Solutions' BRASS.

The co-registered images are displayed side by side with a linked cursor indicating spatial correspondence, or may be overlaid or fused using the gray scale or color display. The spatial correspondence by co-registration between the images of two modalities obtained at separate imaging sessions suffers from positional variations of the patient scanned on different equipment and at different times. In addition, patient motion, including involuntary movement of the internal organs, adds to the uncertainty in the co-registration. Even with the most sophisticated algorithm, an error of 2 to 3 mm in alignment is not uncommon.

To circumvent the problems of positional variations in co-registration of images from different equipment, an integrated system of PET and CT units has been developed by several manufacturers. Similar systems of SPECT/CT and PET/MRI are also available commercially. In a PET/CT system (Figure 2-8) both units are mounted on a common support with the CT unit in the front and the PET unit at the back next to the CT unit. Both units use the same gantry and a common imaging table. The centers of the scan fields of PET and CT scanners are separated by a fixed distance. The axial travel range of the scanning table varies with the manufacturers. Because of the displacement between the centers of scan fields of the two systems, the actual scan field is limited by the maximum distance given by the travel range of the table minus the displacement distance. Various physical features of different PET/CT systems are listed in Table 2.3. A typical PET/CT scanner is shown in Figure 2-9.

The CT unit used in the PET/CT system comprises an x-ray producing unit that transmits an intense beam of x-rays through a patient's body. The

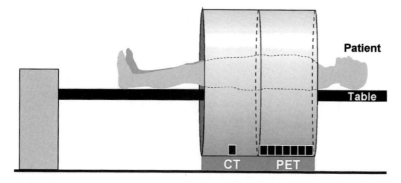

FIGURE 2-8. A schematic illustration of a PET/CT system. (Reprinted with the permission of the Cleveland Clinic Foundation.)

TABLE 2.3. Features of different PET/CT Systems[1].

Company	CTI Molecular Imaging	GE Medical Systems	Philips Medical Systems	Siemens Medical Systems
Model/Product Name	REVEAL XVI	Discovery ST	GEMINI	Biograph Sensation 16—PET/CT
PET Scanner[2]	ECAT EXACT HR+ or ECAT ACCEL	ADVANCE Nxi	ALLEGRO	ECT EXACT HR+ or ECAT ACCEL
CT Scanner[2]	SOMATOM EMOTION DUO	LIGHTSPEED PLUS	MX8000 DUAL	SOMATOM EMOTION DUO
Gantry dimensions, $H \times W \times D$, cm	$199 \times 228 \times 168$	$203 \times 236 \times 109$	$205.7 \times 210 \times 602$	$200 \times 228 \times 168$
Weight, kg (lb)	4600 kg (10,141 lb)	3800 kg (7,600 lb)	3860 (8500 lb.)	4600 kg (10,141 lb)
Patient port	70 cm	70 cm	63 cm (PET) ; 70 cm (CT)	70 cm
Transmission source	CT acquisition	CT attenuation correction	Cs-137 source and CT attenuation correction	spiral CT
Vertical travel, cm	53–102 cm	55–102.5 cm	58 cm	53–107 cm
Patient scan range, cm	156/181 cm	160 cm	196 cm	180 cm
Maximum patient weight, kg (lb)	204 kg (450 lb)	180 kg (400 lb)	204 kg (450 lb)	204 kg (450 lb)
Whole body acquisition time, with attenuation correction and processing	depending on patient weight and injected dose, typically between 7 and 25 min	10–30 min, physician preference	<30 min	15–30 min
Acquisition modes	3-D only	2-D or 3-D	3-D	3-D
Reconstruction time, 2-D mode, 128×128 OSEM-IR	N/A	25 sec (std) 15 sec (enhanced)	N/A	N/A

[1] Most of the data with permission from Reilly Communication Group, publishers of *Imaging Technology News*. Data were obtained from www.ITNonline.net.

[2] Reprinted by permission of the Society of Nuclear Medicine from: Tarantola et al. PET instrumentation and reconstruction algorithms in whole-body applications. *J Nucl Med.* 2003;44:756–769.

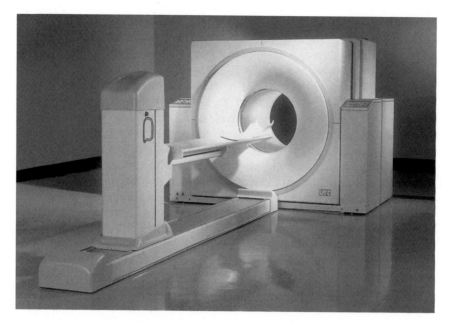

FIGURE 2-9. A typical PET/CT scanner developed and manufactured by CPS Innovations. (Courtesy of CPS Innovations, Knoxville, TN, USA.)

transmitted beams are detected by solid detectors composed of materials such as ceramics, cadmium tungstate, etc. Depending on the design and the manufacturer, a large number of detectors (in thousands) are arranged in an arc form or a full ring around the patient. In the arc form, the x-ray tube and the detector arc are mechanically tied in 180° opposition and rotate together inside the gantry during the study. In full ring geometry, the detectors are arranged in a fixed 360° ring around the patient, while the x-ray tube only rotates. In either case, the x-ray tube projects the x-ray beam through the patient's body while rotating fast around the patient, and the detectors opposite to the x-ray tube detect the transmitted photons, which are stored as counts in the computer. The data are then processed to form a CT transmission image (slice). For scanning the entire body length, the scanning table with the patient has to be translated axially after each slice is acquired. The CT scanner can be single slice or multi-slice collecting data simultaneously for many slices (16, 32 or 64) with different rotation speeds. In helical or spiral CT units, the patient table translates while the x-ray tube rotates around the patient during the examination. This results in a *helical* pattern of the motion of the x-ray tube around the patient, and hence the name. The entire time for a conventional CT transmission scan is only a few minutes at most, and it is much shorter for the helical CT.

The kilovolt in CT units varies from 100 to 140KV and the maximum x-ray energy is 100 to 140keV with corresponding average values of ~70 to

80 keV. The attenuation of the x-ray beam reflects the density of the body tissue of the patient, giving structural information of different organs. An important advantage of a CT transmission scan in the PET/CT system is that the scan data can be used for attenuation correction of the PET emission images (see Chapter 3), obviating the need for a separate lengthy transmission scan in the dedicated PET system. The use of CT scans for attenuation correction reduces the whole-body scan time by 40% to 45%.

The PET/CT scanning is very useful in equivocal clinical situations. A very small tumor is well detected by PET but can be missed by CT. On the other hand, a large tumor with minimal functional deviations may be seen on a CT image, but may not be detected by PET. In both situations, PET/CT would localize the tumor accurately. Overall, accuracy of diagnosis is increased by 20% to 25% when PET/CT is used instead of either alone. It should be noted that at present, while PET/CT whole-body scanning has been highly successful in detecting various oncologic conditions, the application of PET/CT in cardiac imaging has faced difficulty because of the motion of the heart. Ongoing research, however, is attempting to overcome this difficulty.

Small Animal PET Scanner

Animal research commonly precedes clinical use of drugs in humans. The safety and effectiveness of a drug is initially established by studying its in vivo biodistribution and pharmacokinetics in animals. These animal studies using clinical PET scanners are hindered by the relatively poor resolution of images offered by the scanner. For this reason, small animal PET scanners have been developed that permit in vivo studies of PET tracers, providing high resolution of the images. These scanners are small enough to be installed in a small room.

The first small animal PET scanner (Model 713) introduced by CTI/Siemens consists of a single 64-cm diameter ring of 80 BGO block detectors collimated with 7 annular tungsten septa (Cutler et al., 1992). The animal port and FOV are 40 cm and 32 cm, respectively. Each detector module contains a block of BGO segmented into a 6×8 array of crystal elements of dimension 3.5 mm $\times$ 6.25 mm, and the block is coupled to two dual PM tubes. The operation of this unit is similar to that of clinical PET scanners. The sensitivity of this unit is 1.37 kcps/μCi/cc for direct plane measurement, and its intrinsic resolution is 3.5 mm at the center of FOV. However, the need for higher resolution has prompted investigators to build even higher-resolution animal PET scanners.

With the introduction of LSO detectors and fiberoptic readouts of individually cut crystals, small animal scanners with higher resolution have been developed. The microPET developed by the University of California, Los Angeles, consists of 30 LSO block detectors arranged in a continuous ring, and each block has an array of 8×8 individual crystals of dimension $2 \times 2 \times 10$mm (Chatziioannou et al., 1999). There are 8 rings, each with 240 crystals, thus totaling 1920 crystals in the tomograph. The gantry bore is 16cm, and the ring diameter is 17.2cm with a transaxial FOV of 11.25cm and axial FOV of 1.8cm. Each of the 64 crystals in each block is connected to one of 64 individual channels of a multichannel PM tube by optical fibers. Most of the electronics and signal processing are identical to those of clinical PET scanners. The unit has an average intrinsic resolution of 1.58mm and an average sensitivity of 3.92cps/kBq.

Because of the importance of animal work in drug development that later translates into clinical use in humans, further improvement of the small animal scanners is being pursued by manufacturers such as CTI/Siemens, GE Medical, and Philips Medical Systems, and several small animal PET scanners are now commercially available. A small animal PET scanner, called Mosaic PET scanner, manufactured by Philips Medical Systems is shown in Figure 2-10. With the advent of molecular imaging, much progress can be achieved in PET imaging from the use of these improved scanners.

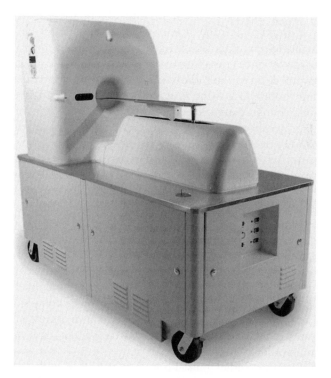

FIGURE 2-10. A small animal PET scanner, Mosaic PET scanner. (Courtesy of Philips Medical Systems, USA.)

Mobile PET or PET/CT

For the convenience of hospitals and clinics that do not have a PET scanner or a hybrid coincidence camera, mobile PET scanners are available commercially to provide PET service to these facilities. PET scanners, preferably PET/CT scanners, along with the control console are installed in sturdy mobile vans. These mobile PET/CT vans move to different client's sites to provide PET imaging services. Because of the scanner's weight and heavy electrical requirement, a concrete pad with enhanced electrical connections must be built at the client site to support the weight of the mobile system. This ensures the correct leveled positioning of the van at the site. The power supply (typically 430V, 3 phase at 60Hz) is provided at the client's site. Also, a generator is installed in the van to run chillers and air conditioning during transportation to keep PET scanners at operating temperatures. Currently, only ^{18}F-FDG imaging is provided by all mobile PET services.

One must obtain a valid license from the state and/or the Nuclear Regulatory Commission (NRC) to operate a mobile PET or PET/CT, providing services to different client sites. The NRC license is required if ^{137}Cs is used as the transmission source, as in the Gemini PET/CT of Philips Medical. In the case of PET/CT, the CT must be registered with the state. A major requirement for the license is to have a letter of agreement between the licensee and the client signed by the management (chief executive officer or designee) detailing the responsibilities of each. Some states do not allow injection of the radiotracer in the coach, necessitating a separate injection room and waiting room at the client's site. Many states may require a sink, changing area, specific security considerations, and fire protection in the mobile van. The van must meet the Department of Transportation (DOT) overload regulations.

All necessary accessories for PET studies, including a dose calibrator, ^{18}F-FDG storage, a wipe test counter, a survey meter, and so on, are kept in the van. The mobile PET van moves daily to different clients' sites according to the schedule made prior to the day of examination. The patient's PET study is performed and the data are processed in the van, while the interpretation can be made either at the van or at the home site of the mobile PET company.

It requires a great deal of logistics in scheduling PET studies at different sites using a mobile PET scanner. The ^{18}F-FDG must be delivered early in the morning, and enough of it should be available to complete the day's schedule. The mobile PET company may have its own cyclotron and radiochemistry laboratory that supplies ^{18}F-FDG to the van, or it may be purchased from another cyclotron facility.

The timing of the studies must be well coordinated with each client to avoid any overlap of schedules with other clients. Overall, mobile PET provides easy access to PET examinations for many community hospitals that are unable to afford a PET scanner because of the cost. However, during inclement weather, the transportation of the van may be problematic.

Questions

1. Describe the general principles of positron emission tomography.
2. Explain why an LSO detector is better than a BGO detector in PET scanning, and NaI(Tl) is least preferred.
3. What are block detectors and why are they preferred to single detectors in a PET scanner?
4. Typical energy resolutions of BGO and LSO detectors in PET scanners are about (a) 10%; (b) 15%; (c) 24%; (d) 5%.
5. The common number of PM tubes per block detector in a PET scanner is: (a) 2; (b) 4; (c) 6; (d) 8.
6. In positron scanners, BGO or LSO detectors are arranged in full or partial rings, and each detector is connected to a number of opposite detectors in coincidence. If there are N detectors in the scanner, what is the maximum number of opposite detectors to which one detector can be connected?
7. The number of BGO or LSO detectors in common PET scanners is of the order of (a) tens of; (b) thousands of; (c) hundreds of; (d) only a few detectors.
8. The number of rings in commercial PET scanners varies from (a) 50 to 100; (b) 5 to 10; (c) 18 to 32; (d) 1 to 5.
9. Explain how SPECT scintillation cameras can be used in coincidence counting. Discuss the advantages and disadvantages of these cameras in coincidence counting.
10. Describe the technique of PET/CT imaging. Why is PET/CT better than only PET in detecting various tumors?
11. PET/CT imaging has the advantage over dedicated PET imaging because of:
    (a) shorter scanning time True _____; False _____.
    (b) higher sensitivity of PET scanner True _____; False _____.
    (c) better localization of abnormalities True _____; False _____.
12. If the travel range of the scanning table is 180cm, and the displacement distance between the centers of the scan fields of CT and PET scanners is 60cm, what is the maximum body length that can be scanned in this PET/CT scanner?
13. The spatial resolution of small animal PET scanners is much better than that of the clinical scanners. Why?

References and Suggested Reading

1. Bushberg JT, Seibert JA, Leidholdt, Sr EM, Boone JM. *The Essential Physics of Medical Imaging.* 2nd ed. Philadelphia: Lippincott, Williams and Wilkins; 2002.
2. Chatziioannou AF, Cherry SR, Shao Y, et al. Performance evaluation of microPET: a high-resolution lutetium oxyorthosilicate PET scanner for animal imaging. *J Nucl Med.* 1999;40:1164.
3. Cherry SR, Sorensen JA, Phelps ME. *Physics in Nuclear Medicine.* 3rd ed. Philadelphia: W.B. Saunders; 2003.
4. Cherry SR, Dahlbom M. PET; Physics, instrumentation, and scanners. In: Phelps ME. *PET; Molecular Imaging and Its Biological Applications.* New York: Springer-Verlag; 2004.
5. Cutler PD, Cherry SR, Hoffman EJ, et al. Design features and performances of a PET system for animal research. *J Nucl Med.* 1992;33:595.
6. Melcher CL. Scintillation crystals for PET. *J Nucl Med.* 2000;41:1051.
7. Patton JA. Physics of PET. In: Delbeke D, Martin WH, Patton JA, Sandler MP, eds. *Practical FDG Imaging.* New York: Springer-Verlag; 2002.
8. PET/CT: Imaging Function and Structure. *J Nucl Med.* Suppl 1, 2004; 45:1S–103S.
9. Tarantola G, Zito F, Gerundini P. PET instrumentation and reconstruction algorithms in whole-body applications. *J Nucl Med.* 2003;44:756.
10. Turkington TG. Introduction to PET instrumentation. *J Nucl Med Technol.* 2001;29:1.

3
Data Acquisition and Corrections

Data Acquisition

PET is based on the detection in coincidence of the two 511 keV annihilation photons that originate from β^+ emitting sources (e.g., the patient). The two photons are detected within an electronic time window (e.g., 12 ns) set for the scanner and must be along the straight line connecting the centers of the two detectors, called the line of response (LOR). Since the two photons are detected in coincidence along the straight line in the absence of an absorptive collimator indicating the location of the positron annihilation, this technique is called *electronic collimation*. In a full ring system, the data are collected simultaneously by all detector pairs, whereas in partial ring systems, the detector assembly is rotated around the patient in angular increments to collect the data. In acquiring the coincidence events, three steps are followed. First, the location of the detector pair in the detector ring is determined for each coincident event. Next, the pulse height of the photon detected is checked if it is within the pulse energy window set for 511 keV. Finally, the position of the LOR is determined in terms of polar coordinates to store the event in the computer memory.

As stated in Chapter 2, in a PET scanner, block detectors of bismuth germanate (BGO) or lutetium oxyorthosilicate (LSO) are commonly used, which are coupled with four PM tubes. Each detector is connected in coincidence to as many as $N/2$ detectors, where N is the number of detectors in the ring. So which two detectors detected a coincidence event within the time window must be determined. Pulses produced in PM tubes are used to determine the locations of the two detectors (Figure 3-1). As in scintillation cameras, the position of each detector is estimated by a weighted centroid algorithm. This algorithm estimates a weighted sum of individual PM tube pulses, which is then normalized with the total pulse obtained from all PM tubes. The weight factor depends on the individual PM tube position in the array. Similar to scintillation camera logistics, the X and Y positions of the detector element in the ring are obtained as follows:

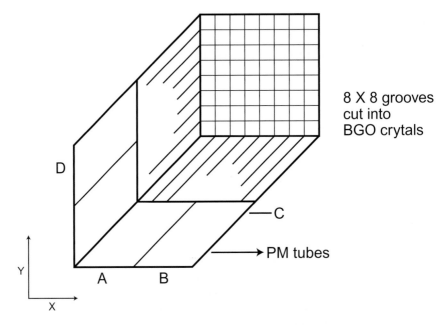

8 X 8 grooves
cut into
BGO crytals

D

C

→ PM tubes

Y

A   B

X

FIGURE 3-1. A schematic block detector is segmented into 8×8 elements, and four PM tubes are coupled to the block for pulse formation. The pulses from the four PM tubes (A, B, C, and D signals) determine the location of the element in which 511 keV γ-ray interaction occurs, and the sum of the four pulses determines if it falls within the energy window of 511 keV. (Reprinted with the permission of the Cleveland Clinic Foundation.)

$$X = \frac{(B+C)-(A+D)}{A+B+C+D} \tag{3.1}$$

$$Y = \frac{(C+D)-(A+B)}{A+B+C+D} \tag{3.2}$$

Here A, B, C, and D are the pulses from the four PM tubes as shown in Figure 3-1.

The four pulses (A, B, C, D) from four PM tubes are summed up to give a Z pulse, which is checked by the pulse height analyzer (PHA) if its pulse height is within the energy window set for the 511 keV photons. If it is outside the window, it is rejected, otherwise it is accepted and processed further for storage.

The last step in data acquisition is the storage of the data in the computer. Unlike conventional planar imaging where individual events are stored in an (X, Y) matrix, the coincidence events in PET systems are stored in the form of a *sinogram*. Consider an annihilation event occurring at the * position in Figure 3-2A. The coincidence event is detected along the LOR indicated by the arrow between the two detectors. It is not known where along the line of travel of the two photons the event occurred, since photons are accepted within the set time window (say, 12 ns) and their exact times of arrival are not compared. The only information we have is the positions of the two detectors in the ring that registered the event, i.e., the location of the LOR is established by the (X, Y) positioning of the two detectors. Many coincidence events arise from different locations along the LOR and all are detected by the same detector pair and stored in the same pixel, as described below.

For data storage in sinograms, each LOR is defined by the distance (r) of the LOR from the center of the scan field (i.e., the center of the gantry) and the angle of orientation (ϕ) of the LOR (i.e., the angle between r and the vertical axis of the field). If we plot the distance r on the x-axis and the angle ϕ on the y-axis, then the coincidence event along the LOR (r, ϕ) will be assigned at the cross-point of r and ϕ values (Figure 3-2B). In a given projection, adjacent detector pairs constitute parallel LORs (at different r values in Figure 3-2A) at the same angle of orientation. The plot of these LORs will be seen as a horizontal row at angle ϕ. When all projections around the field of view are considered, the plot of the LORs at different projection angles and r values will result in the shaded area in Figure 3-2B, which is called the sinogram. A typical normal sinogram is shown in Figure 3-3.

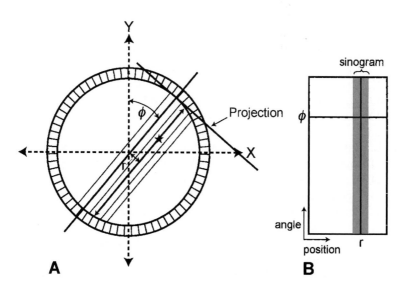

FIGURE 3-2. PET data acquisition in the form of a sinogram. Each LOR data (A) is plotted in (r, ϕ) coordinates. Data for all r and ϕ values are plotted to yield sinogram indicated by the shaded area (B). (Only a part is shown.) (Reprinted with the permission of the Cleveland Clinic Foundation.)

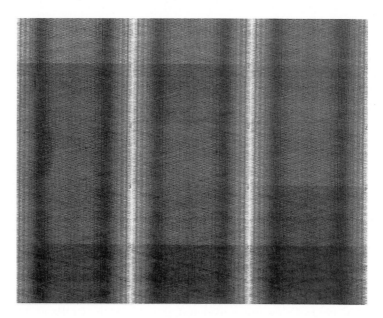

FIGURE 3-3. A typical normal sinogram indicating all detectors are working properly.

PET data are acquired directly into a sinogram in a matrix of appropriate size in the computer memory. The sinogram is basically a 2-dimensional histogram of the LORs in the (distance, angle) co-ordinates in a given plane. Thus, each LOR (and hence, detector pair) corresponds to a particular pixel (or element) in the sinogram, characterized by the coordinates r and ϕ. For each coincidence event detection, the LOR for the event is determined, the corresponding pixel in the sinogram is located, and a count is added to the pixel. In the final sinogram the total counts in each pixel represent the number of coincidence events detected during the counting time by the two detectors along the LOR.

It is of note that comparing raw data acquired in PET with those in SPECT, each projection image in SPECT represents data acquired at that projection angle across all slices, whereas in PET, each sinogram represents the data acquired for a slice across all angles. A set of sinograms from a complete, multislice PET study can be deciphered in the computer to generate a series of projection views that are similar to SPECT raw data.

The data acquisition can be applied to both static and dynamic imaging of an object using the frame mode of data collection (see chapter 4). In static imaging, a frame is obtained consisting of a set of sinograms acquired over the length of the scan, whereas in dynamic imaging, the data are collected in multiple frames of sinograms, each of a predetermined duration. While the static mode is used to display the static activity localization in tissues, the dynamic mode shows the changes in activity distribution in tissues over time.

In dynamic imaging, a gated method can be employed as in the cardiac blood pool gated studies. In these dynamic studies, list mode acquisition of data is helpful providing very high temporal resolution (see Chapter 4). After acquisition, list mode data can be binned into sinograms, and frame durations can be determined. Whereas the static scans are useful to estimate the gross tracer uptake, dynamic scans provide information as to how the tracer activity varies with time at a given site.

Since PET systems are axially fixed, whole-body imaging is accomplished by moving a computer-controlled bed with the patient on it along the axial field, and collecting data at adjacent bed positions. In whole-body imaging, the total scan time depends on the patient's body length and the effective axial FOV of the scanner per bed position. Since the sensitivity decreases towards the periphery of the FOV, the effective axial FOV is less than the actual FOV and it is necessary to overlap the bed positions in whole body imaging. A typical overlap of 3 to 5cm is common, and an even higher value is used in 3-D acquisition, because of the sharper decrease in sensitivity toward the periphery of the FOV. The time for data acquisition at each bed position in whole body imaging is 5 to 10 minutes.

Two-Dimensional Versus 3-Dimensional Data Acquisition

Coincidence events detected by two detectors within the time window are termed "prompt" events. The prompts include true, random, and scatter coincidence events. In many PET systems, in an attempt to eliminate random and scatter photons discussed later, annular septa (~1mm thick and radial width of 7cm to 10cm) made of tungsten or lead are inserted between rings (Figure 3-4A). In some scanners, septa are retractable or fixed, while in others, they are not incorporated, depending on the manufacturers. These septa function like the parallel-hole collimators in scintillation cameras. Mostly direct coincidence events between the two paired detectors in a ring are recorded. Such counting is called the 2-dimensional (2-D) mode of data acquisition. In this mode, most of the random and scattered 511keV photons from outside the ring are prevented by the septa to reach the detectors, leaving the true coincidences to be recorded (Figure 3-4A). The use of septa reduces the fraction of scattered photons from 30% to 40% without septa to 10% to 15%.

Detector pairs connected in coincidence in the same ring give the *direct plane event*. To improve sensitivity in 2-D acquisition, detector pairs in two adjacent rings are connected in a coincidence circuit (Figure 3-4A). Coincidence events from a detector pair in this arrangement are detected and averaged and positioned on the so-called *cross plane* that falls midway between two adjacent detector rings (Figure 3-4A). Instead of two adjacent rings, such cross planes can be obtained from other nearby rings that are

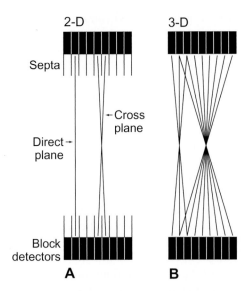

FIGURE 3-4. (A) 2-D data acquisition with the septa placed between the rings so that true coincidence counts are obtained avoiding randoms and scatters. Detectors connected in the same ring give direct plane events. However, detectors are connected in adjacent rings and cross plane data are obtained as shown. (B) When septa are removed, the 3-D data acquisition takes place, which include random and scatter events along with true events.

connected in coincidence. The maximum acceptable ring difference has been ± 5 rings, i.e. a maximum of 5 rings across can be interconnected in coincidence. For an n-ring system, there are n direct planes and n-1 cross planes obtained in 2-D acquisition. Thus, a total of $2n$-1 sinograms are generated, each of which produces a transaxial image slice. While the cross planes increase the sensitivity, they degrade the spatial resolution.

The overall sensitivity (see Chapter 5) of PET scanners in 2-D acquisition is 2% to 3% at best. To increase the sensitivity of a scanner, the 3-dimensional (3-D) acquisition has been introduced in which the septa are retracted or they are not included in the scanner (Figure 3-4B). This mode includes all coincidence events from all detector pairs, thus increasing the sensitivity by a factor of almost 4 to 8 over 2-D acquisitions. If there are n rings in the PET scanner, all ring combinations are accepted and so n^2 sinograms are obtained. However, scattered and random coincidences are increasingly added to the 3-D data, thus degrading the spatial resolution as well as requiring more computer memory. As a trade-off, one can limit the angle of acceptance to cut off the random and scattered radiations at the cost of sensitivity. This can be achieved by connecting in coincidence each detector to a fewer number of opposite detectors than $N/2$. The sensitivity in 3-D mode is highest at the axial center of the field of view and gradually falls off toward the periphery.

PET/CT Data Acquisition

Because of the increased sensitivity, specificity, and accuracy in detecting various tumors, fusion imaging using the PET/CT modality has become the state-of-the-art technique in the imaging field. PET/CT imaging eliminates the lengthy standard PET transmission scan, thus reducing the total scan time considerably. Because of the fact that the patient remains in the same position on the bed, the accurate alignment and fusion of the CT (anatomical) and PET (functional) images greatly improve the detection of lesions. For these reasons, PET/CT scanning is widely used in diagnostic oncologic applications.

Data acquisition in PET/CT is performed in two steps: first CT scan and next PET scan. In a typical PET/CT protocol, a patient is injected with the PET tracer (normally, ^{18}F-FDG) and allowed to wait for 45 to 60 minutes. Waiting for a period shorter than this gives poor target-to-background ratios. After the waiting period, an initial scout scan (topogram) like a conventional x-ray is obtained of the patient during the continuous table motion towards the gantry to define the axial extent of the torso to be imaged. Next, the patient is moved to the CT field of view and a transmission scan is obtained. The CT scan takes only a short period of about 1 minute. During the CT scan, the patient is asked to hold his breath or, if unable, to breathe in a shallow manner to minimize motion artifact. After the CT scan is completed, the bed with the patient on it is advanced inside the PET scanner and positioned so that the PET scan field matches the CT scan field. During the PET data acquisition, the CT scan data can be concurrently used to calculate the attenuation corrections (see later) and to reconstruct the CT images. After the completion of the PET data acquisition, data are corrected for attenuation, and PET images are reconstructed as described in Chapter 4. The CT and PET images are then fused using appropriate algorithms for precise localization of abnormalities. The typical time for the entire protocol for PET scanners using BGO detectors is about 30 minutes, which can be reduced further by using LSO detectors. This is because CT-based attenuation factors can be generated in 30 to 40 seconds compared to 30 minutes for ^{68}Ge transmission scan. A typical study involving the fusion of transverse PET and CT images demonstrating non-small cell lung carcinoma is shown in Figure 3-5.

Several factors affect the PET/CT fusion imaging, namely, patient positioning, truncation artifacts, respiration artifacts, CT contrast agents, and metal implants. In patient positioning, questions arise if the patient should be with arms raised or down on the sides. For scanning the thoracic, abdominal, and pelvic areas, the arms are raised to eliminate hardening of the beam and scatter artifacts. But for head and neck scanning, the arms should

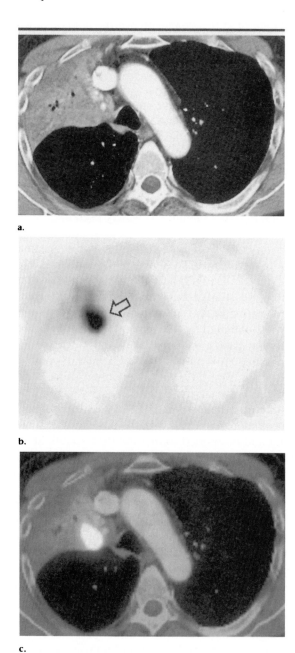

FIGURE 3-5. A study showing the fusion of PET and CT images. Transverse (a) CT, (b) PET and (c) PET/CT fused images showing non-small cell lung carcinoma in the right upper lobe. On PET/CT image, the tumor is accurately demonstrated, which is well differentiated from pulmonary atelectasis. (Reprinted with permission from: Antoch G et al. Non-small cell lung cancer: dual modality PET/CT in preoperative staging. *Radiology*. 2003;229:526.)

be down on the sides so that the area is not affected by the shadow of the arms. Also, the knee should be supported by proper resting aids such as vacuum bags or foam pellets to avoid any artifacts.

Modern CTs typically offer a measured transaxial FOV of 45–50 cm, which is 10 cm to 15 cm less than the common PET FOV. If the patient extends beyond the CT field, which may be the case with large patients, the extended part of the torso will not be reconstructed in CT. There will be no CT-based attenuation correction factors for this part of the anatomy, and the reconstructed images will appear to be blurred by the truncated CT. Careful patient positioning reduces these truncation artifacts in PET/CT scanning. Several algorithms have been developed to extend the truncated CT projections and correct for these effects, but the success is somewhat limited.

Respiration artifacts arise from the mismatch of the images of breathing patterns during CT and PET parts of the examination. These issues have been discussed under photon attenuation later in the chapter. CT contrast agents cause focal artifacts on the PET images due to contrast-enhanced pixels leading to overestimation of attenuation. These effects need to be corrected and are discussed later in the chapter. Metal implants such as artificial joints, dental fillings, metal braces in the spinal region, and so on can cause artifacts in CT scanning, whereas these effects are minimal in PET imaging due to high-energy photons.

Factors Affecting Acquired Data

The projection data acquired in the form of sinograms are affected by a number of factors, namely variations in detector efficiencies between detector pairs, random coincidences, scattered coincidences, photon attenuation, dead time, and radial elongation. Each of these factors contributes to the sinogram to a varying degree depending on the 2-D or 3-D acquisition and is described below.

Normalization

Modern PET scanners can have 10,000 to 20,000 detectors arranged in blocks and coupled to several hundred PM tubes. Because of the variations in the gain of PM tubes, location of the detector in the block, and the physical variation of the detector, the detection sensitivity of a detector pair varies from pair to pair, resulting in nonuniformity of the raw data. This effect in dedicated PET systems is similar to that encountered in conventional scintillation cameras and thus exists as well in hybrid cameras used for both SPECT and PET studies. The method of correcting for this effect is termed the *normalization*. Normalization of the acquired data is accomplished by exposing uniformly all detector pairs to a 511 keV photon source (e.g., ^{68}Ge source), without a subject in the field of view. Data are collected for all detector pairs in both 2-D and 3-D modes, and normalization factors are calculated for each pair by dividing the average of counts of all detector pairs (LORs) by the individual detector pair count. Thus, the normalization factor F_i for each LOR is calculated as

$$F_i = \frac{A_{mean}}{A_i} \tag{3.3}$$

where A_{mean} is the average coincidence counts for all LORs in the plane and A_i the counts in the ith LOR. The normalization factor is then applied to each detector pair data in the acquisition sinogram of the patient as follows:

$$C_{norm,i} = C_i \times F_i \tag{3.4}$$

where C_i is the measured counts and $C_{norm,i}$ is the normalized counts in ith LOR in the patient scan. A problem with this method is the long hours (~6 hrs) of counting required for meaningful statistical accuracy of the counts in the blank scan, and hence overnight counting is carried out. These normalization factors are generated weekly or monthly. Most vendors offer software for routine determination of normalization factors for PET scanners.

Photon Attenuation

The 511 keV annihilation photons originating from different locations in the body are attenuated by the tissue, as they traverse different thicknesses to reach the detector pair in coincidence. If μ is the linear attenuation coefficient of 511 keV photons in the tissue, and a and b are the tissue thicknesses traversed by the two 511 keV photons along the line of response (Figure 3-6), then the probability P of a coincidence detection is given by

$$P = e^{-\mu a} \times e^{-\mu b} = e^{-\mu(a+b)} = e^{-\mu D} \tag{3.5}$$

where D is the total thickness of the body. Equation (3.5) is applicable to organs or tissues of uniform density. When photons travel through different organs or tissues with different μ values, then Eq. (3.5) becomes

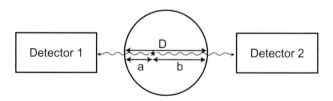

FIGURE 3-6. Two 511 keV photons detected by two detectors after traversing different tissue thicknesses a and b. D is equal to the sum of a and b. Attenuation is independent of location of annihilation, and depends on the total dimension of the body. (Reprinted with the permission of the Cleveland Clinic Foundation.)

$$P = e^{-\sum_{i=0}^{n} \mu_i D_i} \tag{3.6}$$

where μ_i and D_i are the linear attenuation coefficient and thickness of *ith* organ or tissue, and *n* is the number of organs or tissues the photon travels through. Photon attenuation causes nonuniformities in the images, because of the loss of relatively more coincidence events from the central tissues than the peripheral tissues of an organ and also because the two photons may transverse different organs along the LOR. Therefore, corrections must be made for this attenuation of photons in the body tissue.

Note that the probability P is the attenuation correction factor, which is independent of the location of positron annihilation and depends on the total thickness of the tissue. If an external radiation passes through the body, the attenuation of the radiation will be determined by the attenuation coefficient μ and the thickness of the body, as expressed by Eq. (3.5). This introduces the transmission method of attenuation correction, by using an external source of radiation rather than using the patient as the emission source, and the method is described later.

Attenuation Correction Methods

A simple theoretical calculation based on Eq. (3.5) can be applied for attenuation correction based on the knowledge of μ and the contour of an organ, such as the head, where uniform attenuation can be assumed. However, in organs in the thorax (e.g., heart) and the abdomen areas, attenuation is not uniform due to the prevalence of various tissue structures, and the theoretical method is difficult to apply and, therefore, a separate method such as the transmission method is employed.

In the transmission method, typically a set of two to three thin rod sources containing a long-lived positron emitter (e.g., ^{68}Ge, $t_{1/2} = 270$ d), and extending along the axis of the scanner, is attached to the PET scanner gantry. The ^{68}Ge sources on the gantry are rotated by an electric motor around the scanner, exposing all detector pairs to radiation uniformly. In some systems, point sources of ^{137}Cs ($t_{1/2} = 30$ yr) are used. Various transmission sources used in different PET scanners are listed in Table 3.1. Two scans are obtained: a blank scan without the patient in the scanner, and a transmission scan with the patient positioned in the scanner. Correction factors are calculated for each detector pair (i.e., each LOR) as:

$$\frac{I_o}{I} = e^{\sum \mu_i D_i} \tag{3.7}$$

where I_o is the blank scan data and I is the measured transmission scan data. These factors are then applied to all individual LOR counts in the sinogram obtained in the subsequent patient's emission study. However, the blank transmission scan need not be taken for every patient, rather a scan taken at the beginning of the day is good for all patients for the day. Note that

TABLE 3.1. Transmission sources for different PET scanners[§].

	ADVANCE/ ADVANCE Nxi (General Electric)	ECAT ACCEL (CTI-Siemens)	ECAT EXACT HR+ (CTI-Siemens)	ECAT EXACT (CTI-Siemens)	ECAT ART (CTI-Siemens)	C-PET (Philips-ADAC)	ALLEGRO (Philips-ADAC)
Transmission source	^{68}Ge	^{68}Ge	^{68}Ge	^{68}Ge	^{137}Cs	^{137}Cs	^{137}Cs
Source activity (MBq)	370 (×2)*	185 (×3)	140 (×3)	120 (×3)	555 (×2)	185 (×1)	740 (×1)
Source geometry	Rod	Rod	Rod	Rod	Point source	Point source	Point source
Transmissive energy window (keV)	300–650	350–650	350–650	350–650	587–825	595–860	600–720

[§] Reprinted by permission of the Society of Nuclear Medicine from: Tarantola et al. PET Instrumentation and Reconstruction Algorithms in Whole-Body Applications. *J Nucl Med.* 2003;44:756–769.

* One additional 55.5 MBq ^{68}Ge rod is also installed (for calibration only).

the patient's transmission scan must be taken at each bed position during whole-body imaging for attenuation correction.

Using the currently available rod sources of relatively low activity, the above method requires the transmission scan to be taken before the emission scan, and obviously requires a long time to acquire enough counts for good accuracy of the measured attenuation correction factors. Also misalignment of emission and transmission data may result in errors. For example, a misalignment of 1.5 to 2 cm can lead to as much as 30% variation in observed organ activities. An alternative to this approach is to collect the transmission scan postinjection immediately after the emission scan without moving the patient from the bed. This method obviates the need for patient repositioning and hence the need for correction for patient motion and misalignment. Although the residual activity is present from the radiopharmaceutical injection, its value along an LOR is small and the high flux of the transmission source in a small volume along the LOR is enough to mask its effect. However, the detectors must be sufficiently efficient to detect both transmission and emission activities. A further reduction of transmission scan time has been possible by introducing a technique called the segmentation procedure based on the knowledge of prior μ-values of certain tissue types. The measured μ-values from the transmission scans are modified to match the closest allowed known μ-values. This method reduces the transmission scan time to several minutes.

In PET/CT scanning, the CT transmission scan can be conveniently used to make attenuation correction of PET emission data. The CT scan takes a minute at the most, while the ^{68}Ge transmission scan takes as much as 20 to 40 minutes depending on the activity level of the ^{68}Ge source. Thus, it obviates the need for a separate lengthy ^{68}Ge transmission scan. Typically, a blank CT scan is obtained without the patient in the scanner, which is stored for subsequent use in the calculation of attenuation correction factors for patients' emission scans for the day. Next, the CT transmission scan of each patient is obtained and the map of the attenuation correction factors is generated from this scan and the blank scan using Eq. (3.7), which are then applied to correct each patient's emission scan.

The attenuation correction factor depends on the energy of the photons, and therefore correction factors derived from ~70 keV CT x-ray scans must be scaled to the 511 keV photons of the PET by applying a scaling factor defined by the ratio of the mass attenuation coefficient of the 511 keV photons to that of the 70 keV x-ray in a given tissue. This factor is assumed to be the same for all tissues that are considered to have the same mass attenuation coefficient except bone, which has a slightly higher mass attenuation coefficient. The attenuation correction factors are calculated for each pixel and applied to PET emission data. The CT transmission method provides essentially noiseless attenuation correction factors. Figure 3-7 illustrates the effect of attenuation correction using CT transmission scan on transverse whole-body images at the liver level.

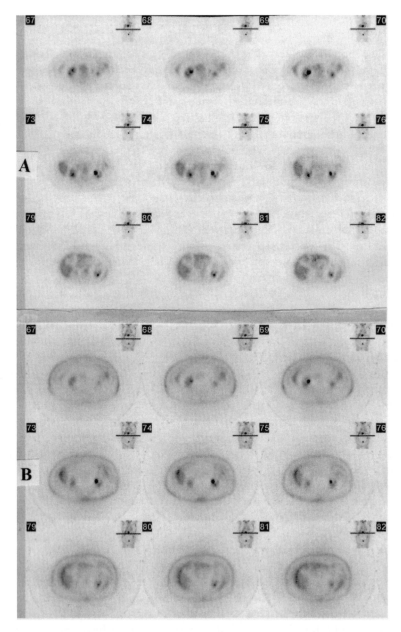

FIGURE 3-7. Illustration of attenuation correction by using CT transmission data on transverse whole body images. (A) Attenuation corrected images; (B) Uncorrected images. Notice that the attenuation correction improves the images significantly showing better contrast and details.

Serious errors occur in attenuation correction factors because of the mismatch between the CT and PET images due to the patient's respiration during scanning. Such errors are maximum when the CT scan is acquired at breath hold with full inspiration (maximum expansion of the thorax), whereas the PET image is obtained at normal breathing of the patient. The diaphragm, the base of the lungs, and the upper pole of the liver are most affected by the breathing artifacts. The use of a multislice CT scanner and a short scanning time (~25s) with breath hold at end expiration may help to eliminate such artifacts.

Understandably, iodinated contrast material enhances attenuation in the areas where the material accumulates, and so contrast-enhanced pixels give an overestimation of attenuation. These pixels are incorrectly scaled to 511 keV and generate focal artifacts in the PET image. Many investigators claim this effect to be negligible on the CT-based attenuation factors, while others advocate avoiding the use of contrast agents altogether. Also, the use of water-based negative oral contrast agents has been suggested for PET/CT scanning to avoid overestimation of attenuation correction factors.

Random Coincidences

As already mentioned, coincidence prompt counts include random or accidental coincidences that raise the background on the images. Random events occur when two unrelated 511 keV photons from two separate positron annihilation locations are detected by a detector pair within the time window (Figure 3-8B). They increase with increasing width of the energy window as well as the coincidence timing window, and with increasing activity (varies as the square of activity, see Eq. (3.8) below). Random events add to the background causing artifacts and loss of image contrast and are more problematic in low-efficiency detectors such as thin NaI(Tl) crystals and in 3-D counting.

The rate of random events is given by

$$R = 2\tau \cdot C_1 \cdot C_2 \tag{3.8}$$

where τ is the time window in nanoseconds for the system and C_1 and C_2 are the single count rates in counts/sec on each of the two detectors on the LOR. Thus, one calculates R by measuring the single count rate on each detector for a given time window, and then corrections are made by subtracting it from the prompts between a detector pair. Note that random coincidence events vary with the square of the administered activity, whereas the true coincidence events increase linearly with the administered activity.

Efforts have been made to minimize random events by using the faster electronics and shorter time window, e.g., BGO system (12ns), GSO and NaI(Tl) systems (8ns) and LSO system (6ns). Still, further corrections are needed to improve the image contrast.

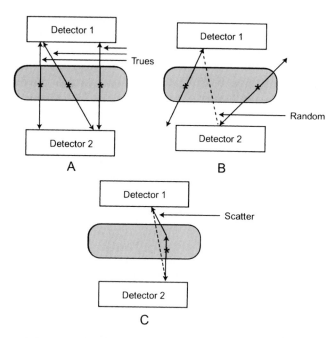

FIGURE 3-8. (A) True coincidence events (B) Random coincidence events detected by two detectors connected in coincidence along the dotted line. The two 511 keV photons originated from different positron annihilations. (C) Scattered coincidence events. Two scattered photons with little loss of energy originating from two annihilation events may fall within PHA window and also within coincidence time window to be detected as a coincidence event by 2 detectors.

A common method of correcting for random events is to employ two coincidence circuits—one with the standard time window (e.g., 6 ns for LSO) and another with a delayed time window (say, 50 to 56 ns) using the same energy window. The counts in the standard time window include both the randoms plus trues, whereas the delayed time window contains only the randoms. For a given source, the random events in both time windows are the same within statistical variations. Thus, correction for random coincidences is made by subtracting the delayed window counts from the standard window counts.

Scatter Coincidences

Annihilation radiations may undergo Compton scattering while passing through the body tissue, and because of the high energy (511 keV), most of these scattered radiations move in the forward direction without much loss of energy (Hoffman and Phelps, 1986). Such scattering may also occur in the crystal itself. Many of these scattered radiations may fall within the energy window of PHA setting for 511 keV photons and may be detected by a detector pair within the coincidence time window (Figure 3-8C). These scattered radiations increase the background to the image, thus degrading the image contrast. The scatter contribution increases with the density and depth of the body tissue, the density of the detector material, the activity in the patient, and the window width of PHA for the PET system. Since both scattered and true coincidence rates vary linearly with the administered activity, the scatter-to-true ratio does not change with the activity. Also, this ratio does not change with the width of the time window, because scatter events arise from the same annihilation event and the two similar photons arrive at the two detectors almost at the same time.

The pulse height window cuts off a large fraction of the scattered radiations, which is limited by the width of the window. In 2-D acquisition, the use of septa in multiring PET systems removes additional scattered events, whereas in 3-D acquisition, they become problematic because of the absence of septa. Typically, the scatter fraction ranges from 15% in 2-D mode to more than 40% in 3-D mode in modern PET scanners.

In practice, the correction for scatter is made by taking the counts just outside the field of view, where no true coincidence counts are expected. The outside counts contain both random and scatter events. After subtracting random counts, the scatter counts are subtracted from the prompt counts across the field of view to give true coincidence counts. This assumes that scattering is uniform throughout the FOV. Other approaches for quantitative scatter corrections are being considered.

Dead Time

When a 511 keV photon interacts within the detector and is absorbed in the crystal, light photons are produced, which strike the photocathode of the PM tube. A pulse is generated at the end of the PM tube and amplified by an amplifier; the energy and the spatial position of the photon are determined and finally a count is recorded. When two such events are detected by two detectors in the time window, a coincidence event is recorded.

The total time required to complete the above steps is defined as the *dead time* (τ), and during this time the detection system is unable to process a second event, which will be lost. This loss (called the dead-time loss) is a serious problem at high count rates and varies with different PET systems. It is obvious that the dead-time loss can be reduced by using detectors with shorter scintillation decay time and faster electronics components in the PET scanners.

In scintillation counting, two 511 keV photons may arrive at and be absorbed completely in the detector simultaneously and, therefore, a photopeak of 1.022 MeV will be produced, which will fall outside the energy window of 511 keV photopeak. If, however, two Compton scattered photons are summed up simultaneously in the detector and the resultant peak falls within the window, then the event will be counted but be mispositioned because of the two unrelated events. These events are called the *pulse pile-ups*, which can cause image distortion at high count rates.

Dead time correction is made by empirical measurement of observed count rates as a function of increasing concentrations of activity. From these data, the dead time is calculated and a correction is applied to compensate for the dead-time loss. Various techniques such as use of buffers, in which overlapping events are held off during the dead time, use of pulse pile-up rejection circuits, and use of high-speed electronics, have been applied to improve the dead time correction.

Radial Elongation

Radiation elongation, also called the parallax error or radial astigmatism, arises from the coincidence events that occur at off-center locations in the FOV. The off-centered 511 keV photons from the patient can strike tangentially at the backside of the detector pair and form a coincidence event (Figure 3-9). As seen in Figure 3-9, the positioning of the detectors by X, Y analysis is defined by the dashed line some distance d away from the actual LOR (solid line), resulting in the blurring of the image due to unknown depth of interaction in the detector material. This effect worsens with the

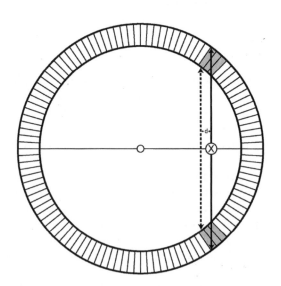

FIGURE 3-9. An illustration of radial elongation. An off-center event (solid line) strikes the back of the detector pair tangentially. The X, Y positioning of the detectors (dash line) is a distance d away from the actual location of the positron annihilation, causing the blurring of the image. (Reprinted with the permission of the Cleveland Clinic Foundation.)

LORs farther away from the center of the FOV and with thicker detector. Also from Figure 3-9, it can be seen that this effect can be improved by having a larger diameter of the detector ring. This effect can be corrected by measuring the light in the front and back of the detector and using the difference to estimate the depth of photon interaction in the detector.

Questions

1. Describe how a sinogram is generated in PET data acquisition.
2. Each pixel in a sinogram is represented by:
   (a) r, ϕ coordinates of the coincidence event
   (b) X and Y coordinates of the coincidence event
   (c) (X, Y, Z) coordinates of the coincidence event
3. The location of the line of response (LOR) is defined by:
   (a) r, ϕ coordinates of the coincidence event
   (b) X, Y positions of the detector pair
   (c) X, Y, Z positions of the coincidence event
4. In whole-body PET imaging, scanning is performed at 5 to 7 bed positions to scan the intended axial length of the body. At each bed position, there is an overlap of 3 to 5cm between scans of two bed positions. Why?
5. In whole-body PET imaging, the overlap of bed positions is larger in 3-D acquisition than in 2-D acquisition. True _____; False _____.
6. The 2-D PET data acquisition is accomplished in a PET scanner by the use of (a) parallel-hole collimator, (b) lead shield, (c) tungsten septa, or (d) concrete.
7. Explain the direct plane events and cross plane events in 2-D data acquisition. What is the total number of sinograms that can be generated in a scanner with n rings?
8. The sensitivity in 3-D acquisition is 4 to 8 times more than that in 2-D acquisition. What are the disadvantages with these high counts, and how can you overcome them?
9. Explain five important factors that affect fusion imaging by PET/CT. What methods are adopted to mitigate these effects?
10. Attenuation of 511keV photons in body tissues primarily affects: (a) uniformity of the image, (b) spatial resolution of the scanner, (c) sensitivity of the scanner.
11. Attenuation of the two 511 keV photons arising from positron annihilation in an organ is independent of the location of the event but depends on the total thickness of tissue the two photons traverse. True _____; False _____.
12. Describe a method of attenuation correction for PET acquisition data.
13. If two 511keV photons arising from annihilation in an organ traverse through a total thickness of 4cm of the organ, what is the attenuation

correction factor? (Linear attenuation coefficient of 511 keV photons in tissue is 0.5 cm⁻¹.)

14. In PET/CT, attenuation correction factors are calculated based on the CT transmission scan that uses ~70 keV x-rays. What is done to correct for attenuation of 511 keV PET photons?

15. Contrast agents used in the CT part of PET/CT imaging cause over-estimation of attenuation correction in PET images. True _____; False _____ Explain why.

16. Describe the method of normalization of the acquired PET data to correct for nonuniformity due to variations in the gain of PM tube, location of the detector in the block, and physical variation of the detectors.

17. Random events can be reduced by (a) narrowing or (b) increasing the coincidence time window; by (a) increasing or (b) decreasing the activity administered, and by (a) widening or (b) narrowing the energy window.

18. Describe the methods for correcting for random coincidences and scatter coincidences in the acquired data for PET images.

19. What are the contributing factors for the scatter coincidences in PET images?

20. Indicate how the true, random, and scatter coincidences vary with activity—linearly or square of the activity.

21. Explain the error caused by radial elongation and how it can be corrected.

References and Suggested Reading

1. Bailey DL. Data acquisition and performance characterization in PET. In: Valk PE, Bailey DL, Townsend DW, Maisey MN, eds. *Positron Emission Tomography*. New York: Springer-Verlag; 2003.

2. Cherry SR, Sorensen JA, Phelps ME. *Physics in Nuclear Medicine*. 3rd ed. Philadelphia: W.B. Saunders; 2003.

3. Cherry SR, Dahlbom M. PET: Physics, instrumentation, and scanners. In: Phelps ME. *PET: Molecular Imaging and Its Biological Applications*. New York: Springer-Verlag; 2004.

4. Fahey FH. Data acquisition in PET imaging. *J Nucl Med Technol*. 2002;30:39.

5. Hoffman EJ, Phelps ME. Positron emission tomography: principles and quantitation. In: Phelps ME, Mazziotta J, Schelbert H, eds. *Positron Emission Tomography and Autoradiography: Principles and Applications for the Brain and Heart*. New York: Raven Press; 1986:237.

6. Kinahan PE, Hasegawa BH, Beyer T. X-ray-based attenuation correction for positron emission tomography/computed tomography scanners. *Semin Nucl Med*. 2003;33:166.

7. PET/CT: Imaging Function and Structure. *J Nucl Med*. Suppl 1, 2004;45:1S–103S.

8. Turkington TG. Introduction to PET instrumentation. *J Nucl Med Technol*. 2001; 29:1.

4
Image Reconstruction, Storage, and Display

Projection data acquired in 2-D mode or 3-D mode are stored in sinograms that consist of rows and columns representing angular and radial samplings, respectively. Acquired data in each row are compressed (summed) along the depth of the object and must be unfolded to provide information along this direction. Such unfolding is performed by reconstruction of images using acquired data. The 3-D data are somewhat more complex than the 2-D data and usually rebinned into 2-D format for reconstruction. The data are used to reconstruct transverse images from which vertical long axis (coronal) and horizontal long axis (sagittal) images are formed. Reconstruction of images is made by two methods: filtered backprojection and iterative methods. Both methods are described below, and Table 4.1 shows the reconstruction methods offered by different manufacturers.

Simple Backprojection

In 2-D acquisition, activity in a given line of response in a sinogram is the sum of all activities detected by a detector pair along the line through the depth of the object. The principle of backprojection is employed to reconstruct the images from these acquired LORs. A reconstruction matrix of a definite size (e.g., 128×128 pixels) is chosen. While the image matrix is in (x, y) coordinates, the sinogram data are in polar coordinates. An image pixel in (x, y) position is related to polar coordinates (Figure 3-2) by

$$r = x\sin\phi + y\cos\phi \qquad (4.1)$$

For each image pixel (x, y) at projection angle ϕ, r is calculated by Eq. 4.1. The measured counts in the projection sinogram corresponding to the calculated r are added to the (x, y) pixel in the reconstruction matrix. This is repeated for all projection angles. Thus, the backprojected image pixel $A(x, y)$ in the reconstruction matrix is given by

$$A(x,y) = \frac{1}{N} \sum_{N=1}^{N} p(r,\phi) \qquad (4.2)$$

TABLE 4.1. Reconstruction methods offered by different manufacturers[§].

Performance	ADVANCE/ ADVANCE Nxi (General Electric)	ECAT ACCEL (CTI-Siemens)	ECAT EXACT HR+ (CTI-Siemens)	ECAT EXACT (CTI-Siemens)	ECAT ART (CTI-Siemens)	C-PET (Philips-ADAC)	ALLEGRO (Philips-ADAC)
Filtered backprojection	Yes (2D/3D)	Yes (2D/3D)	Yes (2D/3D)	Yes (2D/3D)	Yes (3D)	Yes (3D)	Yes (3D)
Iterative algorithms	OSEM (2D)	OSEM (2D) FORE/OSEM	OSEM (2D) FORE/OSEM	OSEM (2D) FORE/OSEM	FORE/OSEM	FORE/OSEM 3D-RAMLA	FORE/OSEM 3D-RAMLA

[§] Reprinted by permission of the Society of Nuclear Medicine from: Tarantola et al. PET Instrumentation and Reconstruction Algorithms in Whole-Body Applications. J Nucl Med. 2003;44:756–769.

where $p(r, \phi)$ is the count density in the sinogram element in the acquired matrix, and N is the number of projection angles. When all pixels are computed, a reconstructed image results from this simple backprojection.

In another approach of simple backprojection, in the reconstruction matrix of chosen size, the counts along an LOR in a sinogram detected by a detector pair are projected back along the line from which they originated. The process is repeated for all LORs, i.e., for all detector pairs in the PET scanner. Thus, the counts from each subsequent LOR are added to the counts of the preceding backprojected data, resulting in a backprojected image of the original object.

Filtered Backprojection

The simple backprojection has the problem of "star pattern" artifacts (Figure 4-1A) caused by "shining through" radiations from adjacent areas of increased radioactivity resulting in the blurring of the object (Figure 4-1B). Since the blurring effect decreases with distance (r) from the object of interest, it can be described by a 1/r function (Figure 4-1C). It can be considered as a spillover of some counts from a pixel of interest to the neigh-

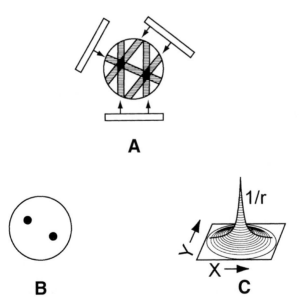

A

B   **C**

FIGURE 4-1. (A) Acquired data are backprojected for image reconstruction at three projection angles (at 120° angle); (B) When many views are obtained, the reconstructed image represents the activity distribution with "hot" spots, but the activity is still smeared around the spots; (C) Blurring effect described by 1/r function, where r is the distance away from the central point.

boring pixels, and the spillover decreases from the nearest pixels to the farthest pixels. The blurring effect is minimized by applying a filter to the acquisition data, and filtered projection data are then backprojected to produce an image that is more representative of the original object. Such methods are called the filtered backprojection, and are accomplished by the Fourier method described below.

The Fourier Method

According to the Fourier method, the measured line integral $p(r, \phi)$ in a sinogram is related to the count density distribution $A(x, y)$ in the object by the Fourier transformation. The projection data obtained in the spatial domain (Figure 4-2A) can be expressed in terms of a Fourier series in the frequency domain as the sum of a series of sinusoidal waves of different amplitudes, spatial frequencies and phase shifts running across the image (Figure 4-2B). This is equivalent to sound waves that are composed of many sound frequencies. The data in each row of an acquisition matrix can be considered as composed of sinusoidal waves of varying amplitudes and fre-

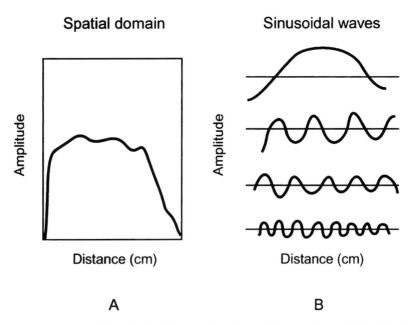

FIGURE 4-2. The activity distribution as a function of distance in an object (spatial domain) (A) can be expressed as the sum of the four sinusoidal functions (B).

quencies in the frequency domain. This conversion of data from spatial domain to frequency domain is called the *Fourier transformation* (Figure 4-3). Similarly the reverse operation of converting the data from frequency domain to spatial domain is termed the inverse Fourier transformation.

In the Fourier method of backprojection, the projection data in each profile are subjected to the Fourier transformation from spatial domain to frequency domain, which is symbolically expressed as

$$F(v_x,v_y) = \mathcal{F}f(x,y) \qquad (4.3)$$

where $F(v_x,v_y)$ is the Fourier transform of $f(x,y)$ and $\mathcal{F}$ denotes the Fourier transformation. In essence, the Fourier transform $F(v_x, v_y)$ of each row in the sinogram of the 2-D projection data is taken and added together.

Next, a filter $H(v)$, in the frequency domain, known as the "ramp" filter, is applied to each profile data, i.e.,

$$F'(v) = H(v) \bullet F(v) \qquad (4.4)$$

where $F'(v)$ is the filtered projection which is obtained as the product of $H(v)$ and $F(v)$.

Finally, the inverse Fourier transformation is performed to obtain filtered projection data, which are then backprojected in the same manner as in the simple backprojection. With the use of faster computers, the Fourier technique of filtered backprojection has gained wide acceptance in reconstruction of images in nuclear medicine.

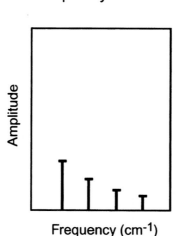

FIGURE 4-3. The Fourier transform of activity distribution is represented, in which the amplitude of each sine wave is plotted as a function of frequency (frequency domain).

Types of Filters

A number of Fourier filters have been designed and used in the reconstruction of tomographic images in nuclear medicine. All of them are characterized by a maximum frequency, called the Nyquist frequency, which gives an upper limit to the number of frequencies necessary to describe the sine or cosine curves representing an image projection. Because the acquisition data are discrete, the maximum number of peaks possible in a projection would be in a situation in which peaks and valleys occur in every alternate pixel, i.e., one cycle per two pixels or 0.5 cycle/pixel, which is the Nyquist frequency. If the pixel size is known for a given matrix, then the Nyquist frequency can be determined. For example, if the pixel size in a 64 × 64 matrix is 4.5 mm for a given detector, then the Nyquist frequency will be

$$\text{Nyquist frequency} = 0.5 \text{ cycle/pixel}$$
$$= 0.5 \text{ cycle/0.45 cm}$$
$$= 1.11 \text{ cycles/cm}$$

A common and well-known filter is the ramp filter (name derived from its shape in frequency domain) shown in Figure 4-4 in the frequency domain. An undesirable characteristic of the ramp filter is that it amplifies the noise associated with high frequencies in the image even though it removes the blurring effect of simple backprojection. To eliminate the high-frequency noise, various filters have been designed by including a window in them. Such filters are basically the products of the ramp filter with a sharp cut-off at the Nyquist frequency (0.5 cycle/pixel) and a window with amplitude 1.0 at low frequencies but gradually decreasing at higher frequencies. A few of these windows (named after those who introduced them) are illustrated in Figure 4-5, and the corresponding filters (more appropriately, filter-window combinations) are shown in Figure 4-6.

F(v)

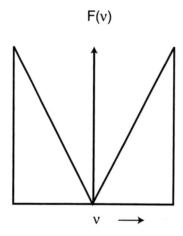

v ⟶

FIGURE 4-4. The typical ramp filter in frequency domain.

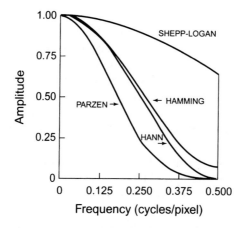

FIGURE 4-5. Different windows that are used in combination with a ramp filter to suppress the higher frequency noise in the backprojection method.

The effect of a decreasing window at higher frequencies is to eliminate the noise associated with the images. The frequency above which the noise is eliminated is called the cut-off frequency (v_c). As the cut-off frequency is increased, spatial resolution improves and more image detail can be seen up to a certain frequency. At a too high cut-off value, image detail may be lost due to inclusion of inherent noise. Thus, a filter with an optimum cut-off value should be chosen so that primarily noise is removed, while image detail is preserved. Filters are selected based on the amplitude and fre-

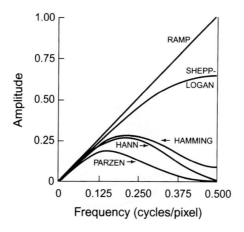

FIGURE 4-6. Different filters (filter-window combinations) that are obtained by multiplying the respective windows by the ramp filter with cutoff at Nyquist frequency of 0.5 cycle/pixel.

quency of noise in the data. Normally, a filter with a lower cut-off value is chosen for noisier data as in the case of obese patients and in ^{201}Tl myocardial perfusion studies or other studies with poor count density.

Hann, Hamming, Parzen and Shepp-Logan filters are all "low-pass" filters, because they preserve low-frequency structures, while eliminating high-frequency noise. All of them are defined by a fixed formula with a user-selected cut-off frequency (v_c). It is clear from Figure 4-6 that while the most smoothing is provided by the Parzen filter, the Shepp-Logan filter produces the least smoothing.

An important low-pass filter that is most commonly used in nuclear medicine is the Butterworth filter (Figure 4-7). This filter has two parameters: the critical frequency (f_c) and the order or power (n). The critical frequency is the frequency at which the filter attenuates the amplitude by 0.707, but not the frequency at which it is reduced to zero as with other filters. The parameter, order n, determines how rapidly the attenuation of amplitudes occurs with increasing frequencies. The higher the order, the sharper the fall. Lowering the critical frequency, while maintaining the order, results in more smoothing of the image.

Another class of filters, the Weiner and Metz filters, enhance a specific frequency response.

Many commercial software packages are available, offering a variety of choices for filters and cut-off values. The selection of a cut-off value is important so that noise is reduced, while image detail is preserved. Reducing a cut-off value will increase smoothing and degrade spatial resolution. No filter is perfect and, therefore, the design, acceptance, and

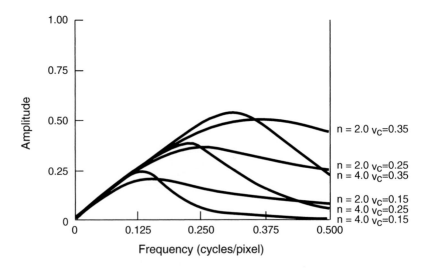

FIGURE 4-7. Butterworth filters with different orders and cutoff frequencies.

implementation of a filter are normally done by trial and error with the ultimate result of clinical utility.

Iterative Reconstruction

In iterative methods of image reconstruction, an initial estimate of an image is made, and the projections are computed from the image and compared with the measured projections. If there is a difference between the estimated and measured projections, corrections are made to improve the estimated image, and a new iteration is performed to assess the convergence between the estimated and measured projections. Iterations are continued until a reasonable agreement between the two sets of projections is achieved. The concept of iterative reconstruction techniques is illustrated in Figure 4-8. Several algorithms have been developed for iterative methods. They differ primarily in the manner in which the projections are computed from the estimated image, the order in which the corrections are applied, and the type of error corrections to be applied to the estimated projections.

Unfolding of the estimated image into a set of projections is considered as the *forward projection*, as opposed to the backprojection, and is accomplished by determining the weighted sum of the activities in all pixels along a line of response (LOR) across the estimated image. Thus, a projection q_i from an estimated image is given by (Figure 4-9)

$$q_i = \sum_{j=1}^{N} a_{ij} C_j \qquad (4.5)$$

where C_j is the counts (activity) in the jth pixel and a_{ij} is the probability that an emission from pixel j is recorded in the ith LOR. The weight, a_{ij}, is equal

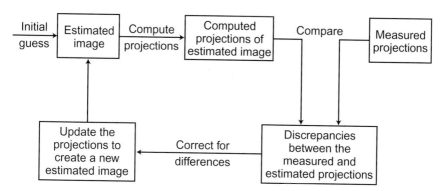

FIGURE 4-8. A conceptual steps in iterative reconstruction methods. (Reprinted with the permission of the Cleveland Clinic Foundation.)

Another algorithm, the row-action maximum-likelihood algorithm (RAMLA) has been proposed as a special case of OSEM requiring sequences of orthogonal projections, which leads to faster convergence than OSEM itself.

3-D Reconstruction

Reconstruction of images from 3-D data is complicated by a very large volume of data, particularly in a multiring scanner. In a multiring scanner having N rings, a full 3-D acquisition would generate N direct (perpendicular to the axis of the scanner) and $N(N-1)$ oblique sinograms (N^2 total) in the absence of septa, compared to $2N-1$ as in the case of 2-D acquisition. Processing and storage of such a large amount of data is challenging for routine clinical applications.

The filtered backprojection can be applied to 3-D image reconstruction with some manipulations. The 3-D data sinograms are considered to consist of a set of 2-D parallel projections, and the FBP is applied to these projections by the Fourier method. The iteration methods also can be generally applied to the 3-D data. However, the complexity, large volume, and incomplete sampling of the data due to the finite axial length of the scanner are some of the factors that limit the use of the FBP and iterative methods directly in 3-D reconstruction. To circumvent these difficulties, a modified method of handling 3-D data is commonly used, which is described below.

A method of 3-D reconstruction involves the rebinning of the 3-D acquisition data into a set of 2-D equivalent projections. Rebinning is achieved by assigning axially tilted LORs to transaxial planes intersecting them at their axial midpoints. This is equivalent to collecting data in a multiring scanner in 2-D mode, and is called the *single-slice rebinning* algorithm (SSRB). This method works well along the central axis of the scanner, but steadily becomes worse with increasing radial distance. In another method, called the *Fourier rebinning* (FORE) algorithm, rebinning is performed by applying the 2-D Fourier method to each oblique sinogram in the frequency domain. This method is more accurate than the SSRB method because of the more accurate estimate of the source axial location. After rebinning of 3-D data into 2-D data sets, the FBP or iterative method is applied.

Partial Volume Effect

In PET imaging, the reconstructed images should depict the radiotracer distribution uniformly and accurately throughout the field of view. However, because of the limit of the spatial resolution of current PET scanners, "hot" spots (structures) relative to a "cold" background that are smaller than twice the resolution of the scanner show partial loss of intensity, and the activity around the structure appears to be smeared over a larger area than it occupies in the reconstructed image. While the total counts are preserved, the object appears to be larger and to have a lower activity concentration than it actually has. Similarly, a cold spot relative to a hot background would appear smaller with high activity concentration. Such underestimation and overestimation of activities around smaller structures in the reconstructed images is called the partial-volume effect (Figure 4-11), and this reduces the contrast between high and low uptake regions. However, this effect also contains the so-called spillover effect due to contamination of activity from the neighboring tissues to these hot or cold areas.

Corrections need to be applied for overestimation or underestimation of activities to these smaller structures in the reconstructed images. A correction factor, called the *recovery coefficient* (*RC*), is the ratio of the reconstructed count density to the true count density of the region of interest that is smaller than twice the spatial resolution of the system. The recovery coefficient is determined by measuring the count density of different objects containing the same activity but with sizes larger as well as smaller than the spatial resolution of the system. Normally, the recovery coefficients would be 1 for larger objects (Figure 4-12). These RC values are then applied to the images of small structures for partial volume corrections. However, the sizes of the in-vivo structures are not precisely known, and so the phantom RC data may not be accurate for these structures. Other methods using point-spread functions of the activity distribution around the object have been investigated with limited success.

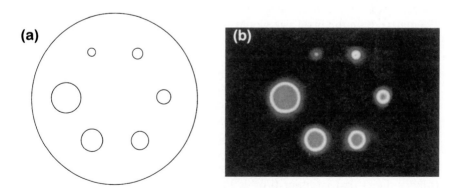

FIGURE 4-11. An illustration of partial volume effect. (a) cross section of a sphere phantom with 6 different spheres, (b) PET images of the spheres demonstrating partial volume effect. (Reproduced with permission from Rota Kops E, Krause BJ. Partial volume effects/corrections. In: Wieler HJ, Coleman RE, eds. *PET in Oncology*. Darmstadt: Steinkopff 2000).

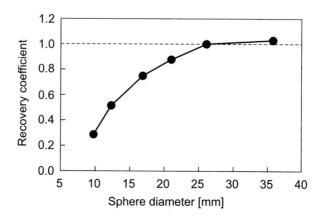

F<small>IGURE</small> 4-12. Recovery coefficients as a function of object size. (Reproduced with permission from Rota Kops E, Krause BJ. Partial volume effects/corrections. In: Wieler HJ, Coleman RE, eds. *PET in Oncology*. Darmstadt: Steinkopff 2000.)

Storage

Reconstructed digital PET images are stored in the computer in the format of a matrix. The images are characterized by two quantities: matrix size and pixel depth. In PET studies, the computer memory approximates the FOV as a square matrix of a definite size that can range from 64×64 to 512×512 with 1026 (1K) to 262,144 (262K) picture elements, called pixels, respectively. The matrix size depends on the type of study and is chosen by the operator. Since the FOV is approximated to the matrix size, the pixel size is calculated by dividing the length of FOV by the number of pixels across the matrix. For example, if an image of 250×250 mm FOV is stored in a 128×128 matrix, then the pixel size would be $250/128 \approx 2$ mm. The spatial resolution of an image is improved by decreasing the pixel size, but is limited by the spatial resolution of the scanner. Pixel size smaller than one-third the spatial resolution of the PET system does not improve the image resolution any more. Thus, for a 6 mm spatial resolution, choosing pixel size smaller than 2 mm does not add to the improvement of the image resolution.

How many counts can be stored in a pixel depends on the depth of the pixel, which is represented by a byte or a word. Digital computers operate with *binary* numbers using only two digits, 0 and 1, as opposed to 10 digits, 0 to 9, in the decimal system. The basic unit of the binary system is a *bit* (<u>b</u>inary dig<u>it</u>) that is either 0 or 1. In computer nomenclature, a byte of memory is equal to eight bits that can store up to 2^8 i.e., 0 to 255 units of information. Similarly, a word of memory consists of 16 bits or two bytes and can store up to 2^{16} i.e., 0 to 65,535 units of information. The color levels or gray shades on the displayed images are affected by pixel depth. Currently 32-bit and 64-bit processors have been introduced, allowing storage capacity of 2^{32} and 2^{64} units of information in computers.

In imaging studies data are acquired either in frame mode or list mode. Details of these acquisitions are given in books on physics in nuclear medicine, and the readers are referred to them. Briefly, in frame mode, digitized signals are collected and stored in a matrix of given size and depth for a specified time or number of total counts. In list mode, digitized signals are coded with "time marks" as they are received in sequence and stored as individual events as they occur. After the acquisition is completed, data can be manipulated to form images in a variety of ways to meet a specific need. This process is time consuming despite the wide flexibility it provides.

In PET studies, the frame mode is commonly used and only occasionally is the list mode employed. The discrete elements of PET images are referred to as voxels, as they represent 3-dimensional volumes of tissue within a cross-sectional image. In the 3-D PET, individual events are recorded in a voxel in a 3-D matrix and the number of total counts in a voxel is denoted by v (x, y, z).

Digital images are commonly stored in the hard drive of the computer. Hard drives with storage capacity of as much as 200 gigabytes (Gb) are currently available. Also, Redundant Arrays of Inexpensive Disk (RAID) provide additional storage in the computer. For long-term storage, a variety of hardware accessories are available. Optical laser disk, magnetic tape, CD, and DVD are common forms of external storage of image data for long periods. Holographic storage is in the experimental stage, but it has the great potential to provide information density on the order of $800\,Gb/in^2$, far exceeding the capacity of currently available disks. For reasons of natural disasters, terrorism, viruses, etc., electronic data vaulting has become an emerging technique for off-site data storage, which provides a means for geographically distant storage and retrieval of data.

Display

Images are displayed on video monitors after the conversion of digital images into analog images by digital-to-analog conversion (DAC) at the video interface between the computer and the monitor. Two common video monitors are cathode ray tubes (CRTs) or flat panel-type liquid crystal display (LCD) monitors. These monitors are characterized by parameters such as spatial resolution, contrast resolution, aspect ratio, luminance, persistence, refresh rate, and dynamic range. These properties are described in standard physics books on imaging, and are not discussed here. It should be noted that the spatial resolution and luminance of LCD monitors are far superior to those of CRTs. These monitors are set in what is called the *workstation*, where practitioners manipulate, view, and interpret images using the computer attached to the workstation.

Display can be in either grayscale (black and white) or color-scale format. Grading of scale in either case is dictated by the pixel values (number of counts in the pixel) in the digital image. The number of counts in a pixel defines the brightness level of the pixel. Thus, in a digital image, the grayscale can be applied to delineate areas of contrast, and when comparing separate images, the grayscale should be kept the same for all images.

Color display of digital images can be obtained by assigning color hues to different pixel values corresponding to counts stored in the individual pixels. In a common color scale, blue, green, yellow, and red colors from the visible spectrum are in order assigned to pixels with increasing counts: blue color to the pixels with the lowest counts and red color to the pixels with the highest counts. Edges of color bands are blended to produce a gradual change over the full range of the color scale. As with the grayscale, the color scale provides contrasts between areas of different pixel counts and thus a means to discriminate between normal and abnormal areas on the images. Conventionally, PET functional images are displayed in color, and CT anatomical images are shown in grayscale. On fusion of the two images, the combination of color and gray scales is quite effective in differentiating the abnormal areas.

Often a grayscale or color-scale bar is shown on the side of the image so that the interpreter of the image can easily differentiate the contrast on the image. The regions of interest (ROIs) can be chosen from sequential images, and time-activity curves can be obtained by plotting counts in ROIs against the corresponding time. Images can be subtracted from one another or can be superimposed, as needed.

PET images can be displayed in transaxial, coronal (horizontal long axis) or sagittal (vertical long axis) views separately, or simultaneously on the same screen (Figure 4-13). On a simultaneous display, a point within an image of the object is chosen using the cursor and three images that pass through that point are displayed. New sets of images are obtained by moving the cursor to a different point along the image. Such sequential screening of images is helpful in delineating the abnormal areas in patients on images.

Angular projections around an object can be computed from the 3-D tomographic data and then displayed in continuous rotation. This results in the presentation of the image data in a movie or cinematographic (or cine) mode whereby a rotating 3-dimensional image is seen on the screen. The relative location of a lesion in an organ with respect to other organs in the body can be easily identified in these movie presentations of PET images.

Software and DICOM

Commercial vendors provide software for acquisition, processing, storage, and display of images specially designed for their scanners. Such software is either developed by the vendor or acquired from a third-party software developer. These types of software use a proprietary format for each vendor, and it is difficult to transfer, store, and display images on equipment

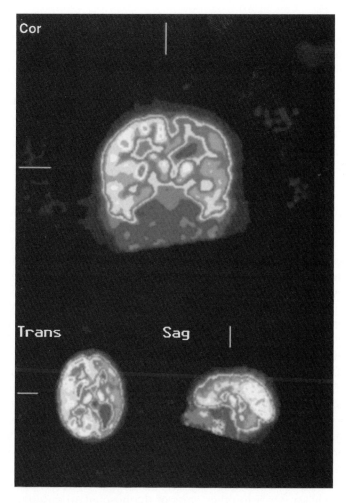

FIGURE 4-13. Simultaneous display of PET images of the brain in transaxial, coronal (horizontal long axis) and sagittal (vertical long axis).

from different vendors. This problem can be partially solved by using equipment all from the same vendor in an institution. To overcome this difficulty, the American College of Radiology (ACR) and the National Electrical Manufacturers Association (NEMA) jointly sponsor a standard format for software called Digital Imaging and Communications in Medicine (DICOM) to facilitate the transmission and usage of medical images and related data among different imaging equipment. DICOM consists of a standard image format as well as a network communication protocol, and specifies standard formats for operations such as Patients, Studies, Storage, Query/Retrieve, Verification, Print, Study, etc.

Currently, major vendors provide software conforming to the DICOM standard, and agree to a commitment to that effect to all customers. Compliance with this standard establishes a common format for imaging systems connecting hardware and software components, and allows interoperability for transfer of images and associated information among multiple vendors' devices. The DICOM standard is particularly useful in the implementation of the Picture Archival and Communication System (PACS), which is discussed here.

PACS

The Picture Archival and Communication System (PACS) is a system for storage of images and transferring images between computers in different facilities through networks. This system consists of devices to produce and store digital images electronically, workstations to view and interpret images, and a network linking computers from different sites. Appropriate PACS software allows the interpreter to manipulate images as needed, at his own location, by retrieving images from other locations via PACS. The introduction of PACS can virtually eliminate the use of x-ray films or Polaroid films for routine interpretation of images, making the imaging centers filmless.

A PACS connects different computers through a high-speed network to share information. This connection can be in a single department using a local area network (LAN), in a hospital using the intranet, or outside the hospital via the Internet. In radiology, it is often desirable to compare CT, MRI, and ultrasound images with those of nuclear medicine studies. A PACS is helpful to provide such comparative studies among different imaging modalities via Web protocols without physically moving to and from different locations of the department. Similar transfer of images can occur through a PACS to other parts of the hospital, to different parts of the country, or even to other countries.

In a radiology department, the Radiology Information System (RIS) is implemented to maintain all aspects of the workflow within the department, from scheduling to billing to reporting. Similarly, hospitals have the Hospital Information System (HIS) that maintains information on patients regarding their demographic data, clinical history, laboratory data, medication, and again, scheduling, tracking, billing, and reporting. A PACS can integrate both RIS and HIS for broader exchange of information among healthcare personnel that will save time and money in healthcare operations. In an integrated system, a referring physician can call in an image of a patient on his computer connected to the PACS, rather than waiting for the hard copy from the imaging department. He can then correlate the clinical findings with the images in the same sitting with considerable saving of time. A schematic integrated PACS is shown in Figure 4-14.

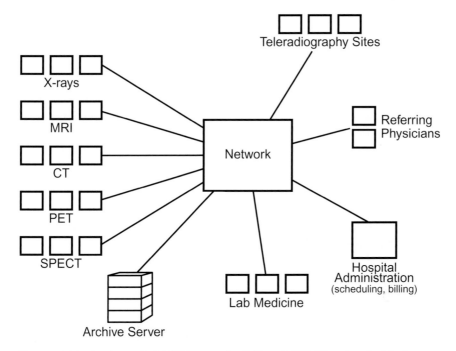

FIGURE 4-14. A schematic PACS integrating RIS and HIS. (Reprinted with the permission of the Cleveland Clinic Foundation.)

A PACS is maintained by a server that provides storage, informatics, etc. for communication among members of the PACS, and also as many workstations as necessary to connect to the server. As already mentioned, at workstations one can retrieve reports and images of patients from the PACS and manipulate them to interpret as needed. A PACS is run by software designed for a particular operating system, such as Windows, Mac OS, Unix, or Linux, although most PACS workstations run on a PC platform. All PACS software can perform some standard functions, but ease of operation may vary. They differ at times in limitation of the number of the patient studies that can be displayed on a monitor screen. The software provides different protocols to access the PACS at the workstation. For example, a protocol may be based on a modality and body part combination such as "CT abdomen/pelvis," or on a secondary descriptor such as "gallbladder stone protocol," or on a subspecialty such as "nuclear medicine." A PACS software should be able to present and interact with all pertinent information for a given patient from different systems, such as the hospital system, the radiology system and the dictation system.

PACS software must address four issues: confidentiality, integrity, reliability, and availability. From the legal point of view mandated by various federal and state regulations, these issues are paramount in the operation of a healthcare institution.

Confidentiality refers to how well private information is kept private, regardless of whether it is a patient, employee, or corporation. Information is available only to authorized persons, and none will be divulged to unauthorized individuals. This invokes the concept of security in the information system. In most cases, security is maintained in the system by introducing an appropriate "user's I.D. and password" format for each eligible user. Recent implementation of a federal law, the Hospital Insurance Portability and Accountability Act (HIPAA), has made it mandatory to insure stricter confidentiality measures in the healthcare system. A PACS should strictly meet this requirement.

Integrity refers to the correctness and completeness of patient information. An error in demographic data or patient medication regimen may result in a fatal condition, which can provoke a legal action. A PACS should provide maximum integrity to maintain a reliable information system.

Reliability refers to the stability of the PACS—meaning the downtime of the system should be nil. If a PACS falters in its operation and encounters frequent failures, it will seriously disrupt the healthcare operation, leading to adverse financial loss. The software should be well written and user-friendly to avoid unnecessary failures of the system.

Availability refers to the timely access to patient information, which can affect the quality of care. Patient data should be entered into the computer on time by the healthcare personnel, as delays can have adverse effects on patient care. Computers and networks must have no or minimal downtime to avoid delays in patient management. A PACS software should address this issue faithfully to maintain an efficient system.

PACS software is evolving over time to meet the challenging demands of healthcare professionals and usually is up for upgrade every 6 to 12 months. Since a variety of factors are involved in the implementation of PACS in a facility, a caveat is in order for purchasing a PACS from a vendor. One should make a thorough assessment of the software prior to purchase. Even though trade shows and demonstrations at professional meetings may offer a reasonable background on the system, one should not hesitate to ask for a visit to sites that have the actual systems that are up and running before making a decision to purchase.

Numerous PACS systems made by different manufacturers are available commercially in the market. Each of these systems is sold as a package consisting of the software and a Web-based server. There are dozens of PACS software companies, such as CTI/Siemens Medical, GE Medical, Philips Medical Systems, Kodak, Agfa, FujiFilm, Dynamic Imaging, Spectra, and Stentor, to name a few, which market the PACS packages that are universally compatible with most imaging systems. Vendors often customize the software to meet the specific need of a customer. All vendors claim their software to be robust, reliable, and user-friendly, with an uptime of more than 99.9%. Even though many PACS versions are applicable to imaging equipment of different manufacturers, it is not uncommon to encounter a few glitches in implementing the PACS of one vendor into a system of a different vendor.

While the importance of PACS is well understood, only 15% to 20% of physicians and hospitals at present use PACS. According to the Institute of Medicine (IOM), an estimated 98,000 Americans die each year due to medical errors, many of which could be eliminated by having PACS because of the quick access to reliable patient information. The IOM is urging hospitals and physicians to adopt electronic record keeping, a measure that could save thousands of Americans. A major drawback of PACS is the lack of a uniform standard for PACS software. To have such a standard, the medical community and perhaps the federal government should come up with a consensus policy similar to DICOM so that PACS can be instituted universally for all concerned.

Teleradiology

A patient's diagnostic images performed at one location can be transferred to different locations by PACS through computer networks. This system is termed *teleradiology* in parallel with telemedicine. Nowadays the practice of nuclear medicine has spread over different geographical regions, and nuclear physicians cover many hospitals and clinics, reading patient scans from distant locations. It is time consuming and impractical for these practitioners to commute to different distant hospitals to read scans. Teleradiology offers a great advantage to these practitioners, because they can read scans of different hospitals from their own locations using teleradiology. For example, on-call nuclear physicians can read scans at home using a computer connected to the teleradiology network through a cable modem, ISDN or DSL connection, or Wi-Fi (wireless) technology provided by the local telecommunications company. Teleradiology has advanced greatly, so much so that interstate teleradiology and worldwide intercountry teleradiology are quite common in modern medical practice.

By virtue of teleradiology, the radiology business groups in the USA are in the practice of global radiology by outsourcing, for example, qualified radiologists in India to interpret imaging scans performed in the USA. This provides a great deal of financial benefit because Indian radiologists are paid less than one-third the pay that their US counterparts get.

Questions

1. Discuss the methods and merits and disadvantages of filtered backprojection and iterative methods.
2. Why are filters used in reconstruction of PET images by backprojection?

3. What is the common initial step that is taken in the reconstruction of 3-D data?
4. When do you apply various corrections (e.g., detection efficiency variations, noise components, random and scatter coincidences, attenuation) in the FBP and iterative methods of image recaonstruction?
5. What is partial volume effect and how do you correct it?
6. A PET scanner has a field of view (FOV) diameter of 20cm. If a 64 × 64 matrix is used for data acquisition, what is the pixel size?
7. LCD monitors are superior to CRT monitors for image display. Explain why.
8. What is the standard format used in software for transmission of images and related data among different imaging equipment?
9. PACS has become the most efficient means of exchanging patients' data among physicians and medical institutions. Specify some important features and advantages of PACS to justify such a unique status.
10. What are the important issues of PACS one should consider in purchasing a PACS software?
11. Most PACS software is PC-based. True _____; False _____.

References and Suggested Reading

1. Bacharach SL. Image Analysis. In: Wagner HN Jr, Szabo Z, Buchanon JW, eds. *Principles of Nuclear Medicine*. Philadelphia: W.B. Saunders; 1995:393–404.
2. Cherry SR, Sorensen JA, Phelps ME. *Physics in Nuclear Medicine*. 3rd ed. Philadelphia: W.B. Saunders; 2003.
3. Cherry SR, Dahlbom M. PET: Physics, instrumentation, and scanners. In: Phelps ME. *PET: Molecular Imaging and Its Biological Applications*. New York: Springer-Verlag; 2004.
4. Dreyer KJ, Mehta A, Thrall JH. *PACS: A Guide to the Digital Revolution*. New York: Springer-Verlag; 2002.
5. Defrise M, Kinahan PE, Christian M. Image reconstruction algorithms in PET. In: Valk PE, Bailey DL, Townsend DW, Maisey MN, eds. *Positron Emission Tomography*. New York: Springer-Verlag; 2003.
6. Defrise M, Townsend DW, Clack R. Three-dimension image reconstruction from complete projections. *Phys Med Biol*. 1989;34:573.
7. Hoffman EJ, Phelps ME. Positron emission tomography; principles and quantitation. In: Phelps ME, Mazziotta J, Schelbert H, eds. *Positron Emission Tomography and Autoradiography: Principles and Application for the Brain and Heart*. New York: Raven Press; 1986:237.
8. Hudson HM, Larkin RS. Accelerated image reconstruction using ordered subsets of projection data. *IEEE Trans Med Imaging*. 1994;13:601.
9. Shepp LA, Vardi Y. Maximum likelihood reconstruction for emission tomography. *IEEE Trans Med Imaging*. 1982;MI-1:113.

5
Performance Characteristics of PET Scanners

A major goal of the PET studies is to obtain a good quality and detailed image of an object by the PET scanner, and so it depends on how well the scanner performs in image formation. Several parameters associated with the scanner are critical to good quality image formation, which include spatial resolution, sensitivity, noise, scattered radiations, and contrast. These parameters are interdependent, and if one parameter is improved, one or more of the others are compromised. A description of these parameters is given below.

Spatial Resolution

The *spatial resolution* of a PET scanner is a measure of the ability of the device to faithfully reproduce the image of an object, thus clearly depicting the variations in the distribution of radioactivity in the object. It is empirically defined as the minimum distance between two points in an image that can be detected by a scanner. A number of factors discussed below contribute to the spatial resolution of a PET scanner.

Detector size: One factor that greatly affects the spatial resolution is the intrinsic resolution of the scintillation detectors used in the PET scanner. For multidetector PET scanners, the intrinsic resolution (R_i) is related to the detector size d. R_i is normally given by $d/2$ on the scanner axis at mid-position between the two detectors and by d at the face of either detector. Thus it is best at the center of the FOV and deteriorates toward the edge of the FOV. For a 6mm detector, the R_i value is ~3mm at the center of the FOV and ~6mm toward the edge of the FOV. For continuous single detectors, however, the intrinsic resolution depends on the number of photons detected, not on the size of the detector, and is determined by the full width at half maximum of the photopeak.

Positron range: A positron with energy travels a distance in tissue, losing most of its energy and then is annihilated after capturing an electron (Figure 5-1). Thus, the site of β^+ emission differs from the site of annihila-

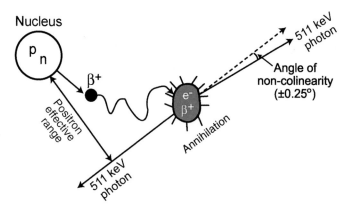

FIGURE 5-1. Positrons travel a distance before annihilation in the absorber and the distance increases with positron energy. Since positrons with different energies travel in zigzag directions, the effective range is the shortest distance between the nucleus and the direction of 511 keV photons. This effective range degrades the spatial resolution of the PET scanner. (Reprinted with the permission of the Cleveland Clinical Foundation.)

tion as shown in Figure 5-1. The distance (range) traveled by the positron increases with its energy, but decreases with the tissue density. Since the positrons are emitted with a spectrum of energy, the positron range is essentially an effective range, which is given by the shortest (perpendicular) distance from the emitting nucleus to the positron annihilation line. The effective positron ranges in water for ^{18}F ($E_{\beta+,max} = 0.64$ MeV) and ^{82}Rb ($E_{\beta+,max} = 3.35$ MeV) are 2.2 mm and 15.5 mm, respectively (Table 1.2). Since coincidence detection is related to the location of annihilation and not to the location of β^+ emission, an error (R_p) occurs in the localization of true position of the positron emission thus resulting in the degradation of spatial resolution. This contribution (R_p) to the overall spatial resolution is determined from the FWHM of the positron count distribution, which turns out to be 0.2 mm and 2.6 mm for ^{18}F and ^{82}Rb respectively (Tarantola et al., 2003).

Non-colinearity: Another factor of concern is the non-colinearity that arises from the deviation of the two annihilation photons from the exact 180° position. That is, two 511 keV photons are not emitted at exactly 180° after the annihilation process (Figure 5-2), because of some small residual momentum of the positron at the end of the positron range. The maximum deviation from the 180° direction is ±0.25° (i.e., 0.5° FWHM). Thus, the observed LOR between the two detectors does not intersect the point of annihilation, but is somewhat displaced from it, as illustrated in Figure 5-2. This error (R_a) degrades the spatial resolution of the scanner and deteriorates with the distance between the two detectors. If D is the distance in cm between the two detectors (i.e., detector ring diameter), then R_a can be calculated from the point-spread-function as follows:

$$R_a = 0.0022\,D \tag{5.1}$$

The contribution from non-colinearity worsens with larger diameter of the ring, and it amounts to 1.8 to 2 mm for currently available 80-cm to 90-cm PET scanners.

Reconstruction method used: Choice of filters with a selected cut-off frequency in the filtered backprojection reconstruction method may introduce additional degradation of the spatial resolution of the scanner. For example, a filter with a too high cut-off value introduces noise and thus degrades spatial resolution. An error (K_r) due to the reconstruction technique is usually a factor of 1.2 to 1.5 depending on the method (Huesman, 1977).

Localization of detector: The use of block detectors instead of single detectors causes an error (R_ℓ) in the localization of the detector by X, Y analysis and it may amount to 2.2 mm for BGO detectors (Moses and Derenzo, 1993). However, it can be considerably minimized by using better light output scintillators, such as LSO.

Combining the above factors, the overall spatial resolution R_t of a PET scanner is given by

$$R_t = K_r \times \sqrt{R_i^2 + R_p^2 + R_a^2 + R_\ell^2} \tag{5.2}$$

In whole-body scanners, the detector elements are normally large and therefore, $R_i(d$ or $d/2)$ is large so that the contribution of R_p is negligible

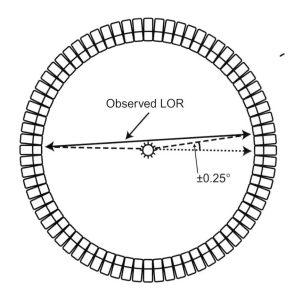

FIGURE 5-2. Non-colinearity of 511 keV annihilation photons. Because there is some residual momentum associated with the positron, the two annihilation photons are not emitted exactly at 180°, but at a slight deviation from 180°. Two detectors detect these photons in a straight line, which is slightly deviated from the original annihilation line. The maximum deviation is ±0.25°. (Reprinted with the permission of the Cleveland Clinical Foundation.)

for ^{18}F-FDG ($E_{\beta+,max} = 0.64\,\text{MeV}$) whole body imaging. For ^{18}F-FDG studies using a 90-cm diameter PET scanner with 6mm detectors, $R_a \sim 2\,\text{mm}$, and assuming $R_b = 0$, $R_\ell = 2.2\,\text{mm}$ and $K_r = 1.5$, $R_t = 1.5 \times \sqrt{3^2 + (2.2)^2 + 2^2}$

$= 6.3\,\text{mm}$ at the center and $R_t = 1.5 \times \sqrt{6^2 + (2.2)^2 + 2^2} = 10.0\,\text{mm}$ at the face of the detector. However, the contribution of R_p may be appreciable for high-energy positron emitters (e.g., ^{82}Rb; $E_{\beta+,max} = 3.35\,\text{MeV}$) and small animal PET scanners (e.g., microPET system) having smaller detectors.

The detailed method of measuring the spatial resolution of a PET scanner is given later in this chapter. The spatial resolutions of PET scanners from different manufacturers are given in Table 5.1.

Sensitivity

The sensitivity of a PET scanner is defined as the number of counts per unit time detected by the device for each unit of activity present in a source. It is normally expressed in counts per second per microcurie (or megabecquerel) (*cps/μCi* or *cps/MBq*). Sensitivity depends on the geometric efficiency, detection efficiency, PHA window settings, and the dead time of the system. The detection efficiency of a detector depends on the scintillation decay time, density, atomic number, and thickness of the detector material that have been discussed in Chapter 2. Also, the effect of PHA window setting on detection efficiency has been discussed in Chapter 2. The effect of the dead time on detection efficiency has been described in Chapter 3. In the section below, only the effects of geometric efficiency and other related factors will be discussed.

The geometric efficiency of a PET scanner is defined by the solid angle projected by the source of activity at the detector. The geometric factor depends on the distance between the source and the detector, the diameter of the ring and the number of detectors in the ring. Increasing the distance between the detector and the source reduces the solid angle and thus decreases the geometric efficiency of the scanner and vice versa. Increasing the diameter of the ring decreases the solid angle subtended by the source at the detector, thus reducing the geometric efficiency and in turn the sensitivity. Also the sensitivity increases with increasing number of rings in the scanner.

Based on the above factors discussed, the sensitivity S of a single ring PET scanner can be expressed as (Budinger, 1998):

$$S = \frac{A \cdot \varepsilon^2 \cdot e^{-\mu t} \cdot 3.7 \times 10^4}{4\pi r^2} (cps/\mu Ci) \qquad (5.3)$$

where A = detector area seen by a point source to be imaged, ε = detector's efficiency, μ is the linear attenuation coefficient of 511 keV photons in the detector material, t is the thickness of the detector, and r is the radius of the detector ring.

TABLE 5.1. Performance data of different PET scanners[1].

Performance	ADVANCE/ ADVANCE Nxi (General Electric)	ECAT ACCEL (CTI-Siemens)	ECAT EXACT HR+ (CTI-Siemens)	ECAT EXACT (CTI-Siemens)	ECAT ART (CTI-Siemens)	C-PET (Philips-ADAC)	ALLEGRO (Philips-ADAC)
Transaxial resolution							
FWHM (mm) at 1cm		6.2 (2D)	4.6 (2D)				
	4.8 (2D/3D)	6.3 (3D)*	4.5 (3D)*	6.0 (2D/3D)	6.2	5.0*	4.8*
FWHM (mm) at 10cm		6.7 (2D)	5.4 (2D)				
	5.4 (2D/3D)	7.4 (3D)*	5.6 (3D)*	6.7 (2D/3D)	6.9	6.4*	5.9*
Axial resolution							
FWHM (mm) at 0cm	4.0 (2D)	4.3 (2D)	4.2 (2D)	4.5 (2D)			
	4.7 (3D)	5.8 (3D)*	4.2 (3D)*	4.6 (3D)	4.9	5.5*	5.4*
FWHM (mm) at 10cm	5.4 (2D)	6.0 (2D)	5.0 (2D)	5.9 (2D)			
	6.3 (3D)	7.1 (3D)*	5.7 (3D)*	6.5 (3D)	6.6	5.9*	6.5*
System sensitivity (net trues) (cps/Bq/mL)	5.4 (2D)[†]	5.4 (2D)	5.4 (2D)	4.9 (2D)			
	31.0 (3D)[‡]	27.0 (3D)	24.3 (3D)	21.2 (3D)	7.3	12.1*	19.0*
Scatter fraction (%)	10 (2D)	16 (2D)	17 (2D)	16 (2D)			
	35 (3D)	36 (3D)	36 (3D)	36 (3D)	36	25	25

[1] Reprinted with permission of the Society of Nuclear Medicine from: Tarantola et al PET Instrumentation and Reconstruction Algorithms in Whole-body Applications. *J Nuc Med.* 2003;44:756–769.

* Assessed according to NEMA NU 2–2001, National Electrical Manufacturers Association; 2001.

[†] Measured at 300-keV LLD in high sensitivity mode.

[‡] Measured at 300-keV LLD.

All other parameters were measured following NEMA NU 2–1994, National Electrical Manufacturers Association, 1994.

Equation (5.3) is valid for a point source at the center of a single ring scanner. For an extended source at the center of such scanners, it has been shown that the geometric efficiency is approximated as $w/2r$, where w is the axial width of the detector element and r is the radius of the ring (Cherry et al., 2003). Thus the sensitivity of a scanner is highest at the center of the axial FOV and gradually decreases toward the periphery. In typical PET scanners, there are also multiple rings and each detector is connected in coincidence with as many as half the number of detectors on the opposite side in the same ring as well as with detectors in other rings. Thus the sensitivity of multiring scanners will increase with the number of rings.

Note that the sensitivity of a PET scanner increases as the square of the detector efficiency, which depends on the scintillation decay time and atomic number of the detector. This is why LSO and GSO detectors are preferred to NaI(Tl) or BGO detectors (see Table 2.1). In 2-D acquisitions, system sensitivity is compromised because of the use of septa between detector rings, whereas these septa are retracted or absent in 3-D acquisition, and hence the sensitivity is increased by a factor of 4 to 8. However, in 3-D mode, random and scatter coincidences increase significantly, the scatter fraction being 30% to 40% compared to 15% to 20% in 2-D mode. The overall sensitivities of PET scanners for a small-volume source of activity are about 0.2% to 0.5% for 2-D acquisition and about 2% to 10% for 3-D acquisition, compared to 0.01% to 0.03% for SPECT studies (Cherry et al., 2003). The greater sensitivity of the PET scanner results from the absence of collimators in data acquisition.

Sensitivity is also given by volume sensitivity expressed in units of $k$cps/μCi/cc or cps/Bq/cc. It is determined by acquiring data in all projections for a given duration from a volume of activity (uniformly mixed) and dividing the total counts by the duration of counting and by the concentration of the activity in the source. Manufacturers normally use this unit as a specification for the PET scanners. The detailed method of determining volume sensitivity is described under acceptance tests in this chapter. The volume sensitivities of PET scanners from different manufacturers are given in Table 5.1.

Noise Equivalent Count Rate

Image noise is the random variation in pixel counts across the image and is given by $(1/\sqrt{N}) \times 100$, whose N is the counts in the pixel. It can be reduced by increasing the total counts in the image. More counts can be obtained by imaging for a longer period, injecting more radiopharmaceutical, or improving the detection efficiency of the scanner. All these factors are limited by various conditions, e.g., too much more activity cannot be administered because of increased radiation dose to the patient, random coincidence counts, and dead time loss. Imaging for a longer period may be uncomfortable to the patient and improving the detection efficiency may be limited by the design of the imaging device.

The image noise is characterized by a parameter called the *noise equivalent count rate* (*NECR*) which is given by

$$NECR = \frac{T^2}{T + S + R} \qquad (5.4)$$

where $T, R,$ and S are the true, random, and scatter coincidence count rates, respectively. This value is obtained by using a 20 cm cylindrical phantom of uniform activity placed at the center of the FOV and measuring prompt coincidence counts. Scatter and random events are measured according to methods described later in this chapter. The true events (T) are determined by subtracting scatter (S) and random (R) events from the prompt events. From the knowledge of T, R and S, the *NECR* is calculated by Eq. (5.4). The *NECR* is proportional to the signal-to-noise (*SNR*) ratio in the final reconstructed images and, therefore, serves as a good parameter to compare the performances of different PET scanners. The 3-D method has a higher *NECR* at low activity. However, the peak *NECR* in the 2-D mode is higher than the peak *NECR* in the 3-D mode at higher activity. Image noise can be minimized by maximizing *NECR*.

Another type of image noise arises from nonrandom or systematic addition of counts due to imaging devices or procedural artifacts. For example, bladder uptake of ^{18}F-FDG may obscure the lesions in the pelvic area. Various "streak" type artifacts introduced during reconstruction may be present as noise in the image.

Scatter Fraction

The scatter fraction (*SF*) is another parameter that is often used to compare the performances of different PET scanners. It is given by

$$SF = \frac{C_s}{C_p} \qquad (5.5)$$

where C_s and C_p are the scattered and prompt count rates. The lower the SF value, the better the performance of a scanner and better the quality of images. The method of determining SF is given later in this chapter. Comparative *SF* values for different PET scanners are given in Table 5.1.

Contrast

Contrast of an image arises from the relative variations in count densities between adjacent areas in the image of an object. Contrast (C) gives a measure of the detectability of an abnormality relative to normal tissue and is expressed as

$$C = \frac{A - B}{A} \qquad (5.6)$$

where A and B are the count densities recorded in the normal and abnormal tissues, respectively.

Several factors affect the contrast of an image, namely: count density, scattered radiations, type of film, size of the lesion, and patient motion. Each contributes to the contrast to a varying degree. These factors are briefly discussed here.

Statistical variations of the count rates give rise to noise that increases with decreasing information density or count density (counts/cm^2), and are given by $(1/\sqrt{N}) \times 100$, where N is the count density. For a given image, a minimum number of counts are needed for a reasonable image contrast. Even with adequate spatial resolution of the scanner, lack of sufficient counts may give rise to poor contrast due to increased noise, so much so that lesions may be missed. This count density in a given tissue depends on the administered dosage of the radiopharmaceutical, uptake by the tissue, length of scanning, and the detection efficiency of the scanner. The activity of a dosage, scanning for a longer period, and the efficiency of a scanner are optimally limited, as discussed above under Noise Equivalent Count Rate. The uptake of the tracer depends on the pathophysiology of the tissue in question. Optimum values for a procedure are obtained from the compromise of these factors.

Background in the image increases with scattered radiations and thus adds to degradation of the image contrast. Maximum scatter radiations arise from the patient. Narrow PHA window settings can reduce the scatter radiations, but at the same time the counting efficiency is reduced.

Image contrast to delineate a lesion depends on its size relative to system resolution and its surrounding background. Unless a minimum size of a lesion develops larger than system resolution, contrast may not be sufficient to appreciate the lesion, even at higher count density. The effect of lesion size depends on the background activity surrounding it and on whether it is a "cold" or "hot" lesion. A relatively small-size "hot" lesion is easily well contrasted against a lower background, whereas a small-size "cold" lesion may be missed against the surrounding tissue of increased activities.

Film contrast is a component of overall image contrast and depends on the type of film used. The density response characteristics of x-ray films are superior to those of Polaroid films and provide the greatest film contrast, thus adding to the overall contrast. Developing and processing of exposed films may add artifacts to the image and, therefore, should be carried out carefully.

Patient motion during imaging reduces the image contrast. This primarily results from the overlapping of normal and abnormal areas due to movement of the organ. It is partly alleviated by restraining the patient or by having him in a comfortable position. Artifacts due to heart motion can be reduced by using the gated technique. Similarly, breath holding may improve the thoracic images.

Quality Control of PET Scanners

In the image formation of an object using PET scanners, several parameters related to the scanners play a very important role. To ensure high quality of images, several quality control tests must be performed routinely on the scanner. The frequency of these tests is either daily or weekly, or even at a longer interval depending on the type of parameter to be evaluated.

Daily Quality Control Tests

Sinogram (uniformity) check: Sinograms are obtained daily using a long-lived ^{68}Ge or ^{137}Cs source mounted by brackets on the gantry and rotating it around the scan field without any object in the scanner. It can also be done by using a standard phantom containing a positron emitter at the center of the scanner. All detectors are uniformly exposed to radiations to produce homogeneous detector response and hence a uniform sinogram. A malfunctioning detector pair will appear as a streak in the sinogram.

Typically, the daily acquired blank sinogram is compared with a reference blank sinogram obtained during the last setup of the scanner. The difference between the two sinograms is characterized by the value of the so-called average variance, which is a sensitive indicator of various detector problems. It is expressed by the square sum of the differences of the relative crystal efficiencies between the two scans weighted by the inverse variances of the differences. The sum divided by the total number of crystals is the average variance. If the average variance exceeds 2.5, recalibration of the PET scanner is recommended, whereas for values higher than 5.0, the manufacturer's service is warranted (Buchert et al., 1999). In Figure 3-3, the average variance between the two scans is 1.1, indicating all detectors are working properly.

Weekly Quality Control Tests

In the weekly protocol, system calibration and plane efficiency are performed by using a uniform standard phantom filled with radioactivity, and normalization is carried out by using a long-lived radionuclide rotating around the field of view or a standard phantom with radioactivity placed at the centre of the scanner.

System Calibration: A system calibration scan is obtained by placing the standard phantom containing a positron emitter in a phantom holder at the center of the FOV for uniform attenuation and exposure. The reconstructed images are checked for any nonuniformity. A bad detector indicates a decreased activity in the image, and warrants the adjustment of PM tube voltage and the discriminator settings of PHA.

Plane Efficiency: The plane efficiency test compares the variations in uniformity of images between planes. After the system calibration is completed, the plane efficiency scans are acquired by keeping the standard phantom at the center of the field. The scans are compared, and interplane efficiency variations are corrected by the computer using multiplication factors to average the plane's responses, which results in uniform images. Note that system calibration and plane efficiency need not be done weekly if the daily quality control data are within the acceptable limits.

Normalization: As discussed in Chapter 3, normalization corrects for nonuniformities in images due to variations in the gain of PM tubes, location of the detector in the block and the physical variation of the detector. This test is carried out by using a rotating rod source of a long-lived radionuclide (normally ^{68}Ge) mounted on the gantry parallel to the axis of the scanner or using a standard phantom containing a positron-emitter at the center of the scanner. The activity used in the source is usually low to avoid dead time loss. Data are acquired in the absence of any object in the FOV. This exposes all detectors uniformly. The multiplication factor for each detector is calculated by dividing the average of counts of all detector pairs by each individual detector pair count (i.e., along the LOR) (Eq. 3.3). These factors are saved and later applied to the corresponding detector pairs in the acquired emission data of the patient (Eq. 3.4). Normalization factors normally are determined weekly or monthly. To have better statistical accuracy in individual detector pair counts, several hours of counting is necessary depending on the type of scanner, and therefore, overnight acquisition of data is often made.

Acceptance Tests

Acceptance tests are a battery of quality control tests performed to verify various parameters specified by the manufacturer for a PET scanner. These are essentially carried out soon after a PET scanner is installed in order to establish the compliance of specifications of the device. The most common and important specifications are transverse radial, transverse tangential, and axial resolutions; sensitivity; scatter fraction; and count rate performance. It is essential to have a standard for performing these tests so that a meaningful comparison of scanners from different manufacturers can be made.

In 1991, the Society of Nuclear Medicine (SNM) established a set of standards for these tests for PET scanners (Karp et al., 1991). Afterward, in 1994, the National Electrical Manufacturers Association (NEMA) published a document, NU 2-1994, recommending improved standards for performing these tests, using a 20 × 19 cm phantom (NEMA, 1994)

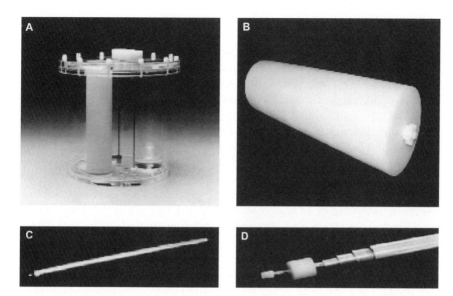

FIGURE 5-3. NEMA phantoms for PET performance tests. (A) This phantom is used for evaluation of count rate, uniformity, scatter fraction, and attenuation according to the NEMA NU 2-1994 standard, (B) This phantom is used for measuring scatter fraction, dead time, and random counts in PET studies using the NEMA NU 2-2001 standard, (C) Line source phantom consisting of 6 concentric aluminum tubes to measure the sensitivity of PET scanners, (D) Close up end of phantom (C). (Courtesy of Data Spectrum Corporation, Hillborough, NC.)

(Figure 5-3A). This phantom is useful for earlier scanners, in which the axial FOV is less than 17 cm and data are acquired in 2-D mode, because of the use of septa. Modern whole-body PET scanners have axial FOVs as large as 25 cm, and employ 3-D data acquisition in the absence of septa. The coincidence gamma cameras have typical FOVs of 30 to 40 cm. Because of larger FOVs and high count rates in 3-D mode, the NU 2-1994 phantom may not be accurately applied for some tests in some scanners, and a new NU 2-2001 standard has been published by NEMA in 2001 (NEMA, 2001). The phantom used measures 70 cm long compared to 19 cm for the NU 2-1994 phantom (Figure 5-3B). While the NU 2-1994 phantom is still used for some parameters and in earlier scanners, the NU 2-2001 standard is employed to measure several parameters (e.g., sensitivity) in modern whole-body scanners and coincidence gamma cameras. Daube-Witherspoon et al. (2002) have reported the methods of performing these tests based on the NEMA NU 2-2001 standard. The following is a brief description of these tests for some important parameters based on this article and the methods of NEMA NU 2-2001 standard. One should refer to Daube-Witherspoon et al. (2002), NU 2-1994 and NU 2-2001 standards of NEMA for details. Various pertinent parameters for PET scanners from different manufacturers are given in Table 5.1. Note that the table contains data based on both standards.

Spatial Resolution

The spatial resolution of a PET scanner is determined by the full width at half maximum (FWHM) of point-spread-functions (PSF) obtained from measurement of activity distribution from a point source. The spatial resolution can be transverse radial, transverse tangential, and axial, and these values are given in Table 5.1 for scanners from different manufacturers.

The spatial resolution is measured by using six point sources of ^{18}F activity contained in glass capillary in a small volume of less than 1cc (Daube-Witherspoon et al., 2002). For axial resolutions, two positions—at the center of the axial FOV and at $1/4^{th}$ of axial FOV—are chosen (Figure 5-4). At each axial position, three point sources are placed at $x = 0, y = 1$cm (to avoid too many sampling of LORs), $x = 10$cm, $y = 0$, and $x = 0, y = 10$cm. Data are collected for all six positions and from reconstructed image data, PSFs are obtained in X, Y, and Z directions for each point source at each axial position. The FWHMs are determined from the width at 50% of the peak of each PSF, totaling 18 in number. Related FWHMs are combined and then averaged for the two axial positions to give the transverse radial, transverse tangential and axial resolutions. Transverse resolution worsens as the source is moved away from the center of the FOV (Figure 5-5), i.e., the resolution is best at the center and deteriorates toward the periphery of the scanner.

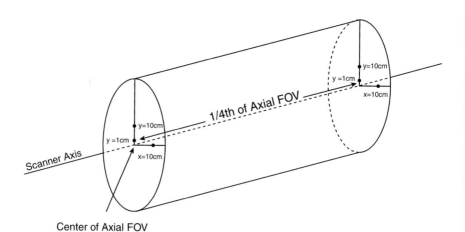

FIGURE 5-4. Arrangement of 6-point sources in the measurement of spatial resolution. Three sources are positioned at the center of the axial FOV and 3 sources are positioned at $1/4^{th}$ of the axial FOB away from the center. At each position, sources are placed on the positions indicated in a transverse plane perpendicular to the scanner axis. (Reprinted with the permission of the Cleveland Clinic Foundation.)

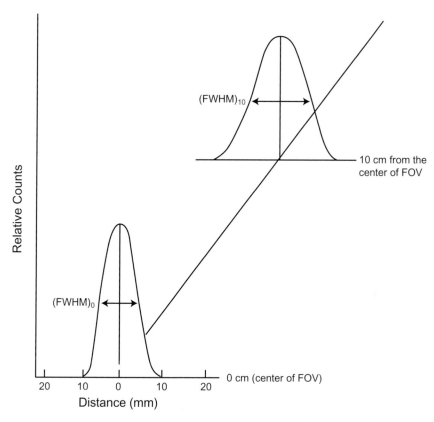

FIGURE 5-5. Point spread functions (PSF) at 0 and 10cm from the center of the FOV. The transverse resolution (FWHM) is best at the center and worsens both radially and axially across the FOV. (Reprinted with the permission of the Cleveland Clinic Foundation.)

Scatter Fraction

Scattered radiations add noise to the reconstructed image, and the contribution varies with different PET scanners. Normally the test is performed with a very high activity source counted over a period of time, from which high activity data are used for determination of random events and count losses (see later) and low activity data for scatter fraction. A narrow line source made of 70cm long plastic tubing and filled with high activity of ^{18}F is inserted into a 70×20cm cylindrical polyethylene phantom through an axial hole made at a radial distance of 4.5cm and parallel to the central axis of the phantom (Figure 5-3B). The phantom is placed at the center both axially and radially on the scan table such that the source is closest to the patient table, since the line source and the bed position affect the measured results.

Data are acquired over time until dead time count losses and random events are reduced to less than 1% of the true rates. These low activity data are used to form sinograms for calculation of scatter fractions. A sinogram profile of an extended diameter of 24cm (4cm larger than the phantom) is used, because the FOV varies with different scanners. Each projection in the sinogram is shifted so that the peak of the projection is aligned with the center of the sinogram (line source image). This produces a sum projection with a counts density distribution around the maximum counts (peak) at the center of the sinogram (NEMA, 2001). It is arbitrarily assumed that all true events including some scatter lie within a 4-cm-wide strip centered in each sinogram of the line source and there are no true events but scatter events beyond ±2cm from the center of the sinogram. Thus the total counts C_T is the area under the peak that includes true events and scatter events plus scatter events outside the peak. The scattered events under the peak are then estimated by taking the average of the pixel counts at ±2cm positions from the center and multiplying the average with the number of pixels along the 4-cm strip. The product is added to the counts in pixels outside the peak to give total scatter events for the slice. For better statistical accuracy, several acquisitions are made, and the total counts and scatter counts of the corresponding slices are separately summed for all acquisitions. Note that the total counts, C_T, has no or negligible random counts. If C_S and C_T are the scatter counts and total counts, respectively, for a slice, then the scatter fraction SF_i for the slice is given by Eq. (5.5) as

$$SF_i = C_S/C_T \tag{5.7}$$

The system scatter fraction SF is calculated from the weighted average of the SF_i values of all slices. The true count rate R_{true} for a slice is calculated as

$$R_{true} = (C_T - C_S)/t \tag{5.8}$$

where t is the total time of acquisition.

Sensitivity

The sensitivity is a measure of counting efficiency of a PET scanner and is expressed in count rate (normally, cps) per unit activity concentration (normally, MBq or μCi per cc). The NU 2-1994 standard using the 20×19cm phantom underestimates the sensitivity of larger whole-body scanners. The phantom recommended in the NU 2-2001 standard also is too large (70×20cm) and impractical to fill and handle radioactivity. Instead, a 70-cm-long plastic tube filled with a known amount (A_{cal}) of a radionuclide is used (Figure 5-3C, D) (Daube-Whitherspoon et al., 2002). The level of activity is kept low so as to have negligible random events and count loss. The source is encased in metal sleeves of various thicknesses and suspended at the center of the transverse FOV in parallel to the axis of the scanner in such a way that the supporting unit stays outside the FOV.

Successive data are collected in sinograms using five metal sleeves and an energy window of 410 to 665 keV. Duration of acquisition and total counts in the slice are recorded for each sleeve, from which the count rate is calculated. The count rates are corrected for decay to the time of calibration of radioactivity and then summed for all slices to give the total count rate for each sleeve. Next, the natural logarithm of the measured total count rate (R_i) is plotted as a function of sleeve thickness. After fitting of the data by linear regression, the extrapolated count rate (R_0) with no metal sleeve (attenuation correction) is obtained. The system sensitivity S is given by

$$S = R_0 / A_{cal} \tag{5.9}$$

where A_{cal} is the calibrated activity added to the tubing. The sensitivity is given in either $kcps/\mu Ci/cc$ or $cps/MBq/cc$. The measurement of sensitivity is repeated with the source placed radially at 10 cm from the center of the transverse FOV. The system sensitivity of commercial PET scanners for 0 cm position is given in Table 5.1.

Count Rate Losses and Random Coincidences

To characterize the count rate behavior of a PET scanner at high activity, random events, noise equivalent count rate, and dead time loss are determined as a function of activity. The activity source is the same as described above under Scatter Fraction in this chapter. A high activity source of ^{18}F is used to acquire the sinogram and data are collected using an energy window of 410 to 665 keV until the activity level is low enough to consider random events and dead time count losses to be negligible. The total counts are obtained from each high activity sinogram, which comprise true, random and scatter events. The total count rate R_T is obtained by dividing the total counts by the duration of acquisition. As in scatter fraction experiment, the low activity data are used to calculate the scatter fraction SF_i and the true count rate R_{true} for each slice (Eqs. 5.7 and 5.8). The random count rate R_r for each slice is then calculated by (Daube-Witherspoon et al., 2002)

$$R_r = R_T - [R_{true}/(1 - SF_i)] \tag{5.10}$$

The system random count rate is calculated by summing R_r values for all slices.

The noise equivalent count rate ($NECR$) for each slice is computed by Eq. (5.4) as

$$NECR = (R_{true})^2 / R_T \tag{5.11}$$

The system $NECR$ is computed as the sum of all $NECR$s over all slices.

The percent dead time count loss ($\%DT$) as function of activity is calculated by

$$\%DT = (1 - R/R_{extrap}) \times 100 \qquad (5.12)$$

where R_{extrap} is the count rate extrapolated from the low activity data to the time when the total count rate R_T is measured, and R is the true count rate (equal to R_T corrected for scatter and random events).

Questions

1. The typical transaxial resolution at 1 cm of a PET scanner ranges between (A) 14 and 16 mm (B) 3 and 4 cm (C) 4 and 7 mm.
2. What are the common factors that affect the spatial resolution of a PET scanner? Out of these, which one is most predominant?
3. The transverse resolution is worse at the center of the FOV than away from the center. True _____; False _____.
4. The axial resolution of a scanner is its ability to differentiate two points on an image along the axis of the scanner. True _____; False _____.
5. If the detector size is 8 mm, what is the expected approximate spatial resolution for ^{18}F-FDG PET images at the center of the FOV?
6. The maximum positron energy for ^{18}F is 0.64 MeV and for ^{82}Rb is 3.35 MeV. Which radiopharmaceutical would provide better spatial resolution?
7. Non-colinearity is a factor that affects the spatial resolution of a PET scanner. How is it affected by the diameter of the detector ring? For a 90 cm diameter detector ring, what is the value of the non-colinearity component in the overall spatial resolution?
8. Describe the method of measuring transverse radial, transverse tangential, and axial spatial resolutions of a PET scanner.
9. Define the sensitivity of a PET scanner and discuss the important parameters that affect the sensitivity.
10. Scanner 1 has twice the ring diameter of scanner 2. The ratio of sensitivities of scanner 1 to scanner 2 is:
    (A) 0.75
    (B) 0.67
    (C) 0.25
11. The sensitivity in 3-D acquisition is 4 to 8 times higher than in 2-D acquisition. Why?
12. The overall sensitivities of PET scanners in 2-D mode are:
    (a) 1 to 2%
    (b) 3 to 5%
    (c) 0.2 to 0.5%

and in 3-D mode:
(a) 20 to 30%
(b) 2 to 10%
(c) 35 to 45%
13. Scanner 1 has the detectors of size 3 mm, and scanner 2 has the detectors of size 6 mm. Assuming that all detectors are squares and all other parameters are the same, the sensitivity of scanner 1 is: (A) half; (B) one-tenth; or (C) one-fourth of scanner 2.
14. Describe the methods of daily and weekly quality control tests.
15. Explain why and how normalization of PET acquisition data is carried out.
16. What are acceptance tests? Describe the methods of determining sensitivity and scatter fraction for a PET scanner.
17. The noise equivalent count rate ($NECR$) is proportional to the signal-to-noise in the reconstructed image. True _____; False _____.
18. The sensitivity of a scanner increases with (A) the size of the detector in the ring True _____; False _____; (B) with the diameter of the detector ring True _____; False _____.
19. Scanner 1 has the individual detector size of 36 mm² and scanner 2 has the detector size of 60 mm². Scanner 1 has (A) 30%; (B) 60%; (C) 1.7 times the sensitivity of scanner 2.
20. Define contrast of an image. Elucidate the different factors that affect the contrast.

References and Suggested Reading

1. Budinger TF. PET instrumentation: what are the limits? *Semin Nucl Med.* 1998;28:247.
2. Brix G, Zaers J, Adam LE, et al. Performance evaluation of a whole-body PET scanner using the NEMA protocol. *J Nucl Med.* 1997;38:1614.
3. Buchert R, Bohuslavizki UH, Mester J, et al. Quality assurance in PET: Evaluation of the clinical relevance of detector defects. *J Nucl Med.* 1999; 40:1657.
4. Daube-Witherspoon ME, Karp JS, Casey ME, et al. PET performance measurement using the NEMA NU 2-2001 standard. *J Nucl Med.* 2002;43:1398.
5. Huesman RH. The effects of a finite number of projection angles and finite lateral sampling of projections on the propagation of statistical errors in transverse section reconstruction. *Phys Med Biol.* 1977;22:511.
6. Karp JS, Daube-Witherspoon ME, Hoffman EJ, et al. Performance standards in positron emission tomography. *J Nucl Med.* 1991;32:2342.
7. Kearfott K. Sinograms and diagnostic tools for the quality assurance of a positron emission tomograph. *J Nucl Med Technol.* 1989;17:83.
8. Keim P. An overview of PET quality assurance procedures: Part 1. *J Nucl Med Technol.* 1994;22:27.
9. Moses WW, Derenzo SE. Empirical observation of performance degradation in positron emission tomographs utilizing block detectors. *J Nucl Med.* 1993; 34:101P.

10. National Electrical Manufacturers Association. NEMA Standards Publications NU 2-1994. *Performance Measurements of Positron Emission Tomographs.* Washington DC: National Electrical Manufacturers Association; 1994.
11. National Electrical Manufacturers Association. NEMA Standard Publication NU 2-2001. *Performance Measurements of Positron Emission Tomographs.* Rosslyn, VA: National Electrical Manufacturers Association; 2001.
12. Tarantola G, Zito F, Gerundini P. PET instrumentation and reconstruction algorithms in whole-body applications. J Nucl Med 2003;44:756.

6
Cyclotron and Production of PET Radionuclides

More than 3000 nuclides are known, of which approximately 270 are stable and the remainder are radioactive. The majority of radionuclides are artificially produced in the cyclotron and reactor. In PET technology, only positron-emitting radionuclides are required, and only a few positron emitters of all radionuclides have been suitably utilized in the clinical studies. These radionuclides include ^{11}C, ^{13}N, ^{18}F, ^{15}O, etc. and are produced in the cyclotron. The operation of a cyclotron and the production of useful positron emitters are described below.

Cyclotron Operation

In a cyclotron (Figure 6-1), charged particles (S) are accelerated in circular paths within the two D-shaped hollow metallic electrodes called the *dees* (A and B) under vacuum by means of an electromagnetic field. Charged particles can be either positive ions (e.g. proton, deuteron, α particle) or negative ions (e.g. negatively charged hydrogen atom, H⁻). The following is a description of a cyclotron to accelerate H⁻ particles (negative ion cyclotrons).

The ions are obtained from an ion source (S) positioned at the center of the cyclotron. The ion source is a small chamber located between two negative high-voltage (V) (1 to 3kV) tantalum cathodes. The hydrogen gas flows (4 to 10mL/min) into the chamber. Electrons emitted from the cathodes and constrained by the magnetic field of the main magnet interact with the hydrogen atoms to form a plasma in the chamber that consists of 3 entities: protons, negatively charged hydrogen atoms H⁻, and neutral hydrogen atoms. In some cyclotrons, the gas is ionized by applying 20kV DC, producing proton and H⁻. Protons or negative hydrogen ions (H⁻) are pulled out of the ion source chamber through a narrow slit by the electrostatic force depending on the polarity of the dees.

The two dees (A and B) are half-pie-shaped, troughlike, hollow copper structures connected to an alternating high-voltage (30KV) oscillator oper-

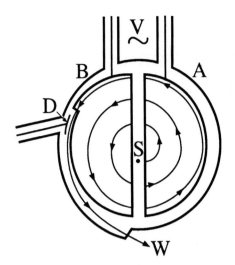

FIGURE 6-1. A schematic illustration of a cyclotron: V, alternating voltage; S, ion source; A and B, dees under vacuum; D, carbon foil stripper; W, window.

ating at radiofrequencies of 16 to 25 MHz and are positioned between the two poles of an electromagnet. In some cyclotrons, there are four dees, which look like a quarter of a pie. The inside of the dees is kept at extremely high vacuum (10^{-6} mtorr for positive ions and 10^{-7} mtorr for negative ions). Since H$^-$ can lose its electrons on interaction with any molecule inside the dee, such high vacuum is essential in negative ion cyclotrons, which is tenfold higher than in positive ion cyclotrons. Charged ions are attracted toward a dee with an opposite charge during the cycle of oscillating radiofrequency voltage waveforms and pass into the hollow dee. While in the dee, ions do not experience any electrical field, but are subjected to a magnetic field provided by a large electromagnet (up to 2 tesla). Under the magnetic field, the path of the ions bends such that as the ions reach the edge of the dee, the polarity of the dee is changed. At this moment, the ions are repelled by the dee and also attracted toward the opposite dee, thus gaining more kinetic energy to accelerate. The radiofrequency is so synchronized that every time the ions cross the dee intersection, the polarity of the dee is changed and the ions gain energy and travel in a larger trajectory in the dee. For a particular cyclotron, the energy of the ions depends on the radius of the cyclotron, magnetic field and charge and mass of the ion. Thus, the kinetic energy (K.E.) of the ion is given by

$$K.E. = \frac{(qMr)^2}{2m} \qquad (6.1)$$

where q is the charge of the particle, M is the magnetic field in gauss, r is the radius of the cyclotron, and m is the mass of the particle.

Since negative H$^-$ ions do not interact with the nuclei of the target and positive ions do, a 2- to 5-μm-thick <4 cm in diameter carbon foil (D) is inserted vertically inside the cyclotron to strip two electrons to produce positive ions (i.e. protons), which then can cause nuclear reactions in target nuclei. The positioning of the carbon foil is computer-controlled. By using two carbon-stripping foils and stripping only a portion of the beam through each one, the beam can be split into two that are aimed at two separate targets simultaneously. Under the influence of the electromagnet, the protons then spiral out through the window (W) as an external beam. The kinetic energy of the accelerated particles can vary from a few MeV to several billion electron volts (GeV), depending on the size and design of the cyclotron. For a given cyclotron, the external beam energy remains constant, whereas the internal beam energy varies radially inside the cyclotron. This variable energy of the particles can be utilized by placing a probe at different radial positions. Various particles, namely, α particle, proton, deuteron, ^{3}He, and a few heavy ions can be accelerated depending on the design of the cyclotron. The operation of cyclotrons is mostly automatic with minimal manual input and is controlled by the computer.

Medical Cyclotron

Medical cyclotrons are compact cyclotrons that are primarily used to produce short-lived, positron-emitting radionuclides used for PET imaging. Most of the clinically useful positron emitters are formed by nuclear reactions with low-energy particles and hence the compact cyclotrons. These are commercially available and can be installed in a relatively small space. Moreover, in medical cyclotrons, negative hydrogen ions (H$^-$) are commonly accelerated, because unlike in positive ion cyclotrons, the housing of the cyclotron does not become radioactive in negative ion cyclotrons. Also, the beam can be split by two carbon-stripping foils so that two targets can be irradiated simultaneously. Whereas the particle energy may be in the range of a billion electron volts in high-energy cyclotrons, the typical energy of the protons or H$^-$ particles in medical cyclotrons ranges between 10 and 18 MeV. In some medical cyclotrons, both deuterons and H$^-$ particles can be accelerated interchangeably by switching the ion sources between deuterium and hydrogen. Shielding is a major concern for cyclotron installation. Whereas, in high-energy cyclotrons, shielding is achieved mostly by thick concrete walls and with large separation between the walls and the cyclotron, medical cyclotrons are mostly self-shielded with lead blocks because of their compact nature. The shielding commonly consists of four lead block quadrants supported on coasters that wheel in and out for closing and opening of the quadrants for easy access to the cyclotron for maintenance. The operation of a medical cyclotron is a turn-key type and computer controlled, and a technologist with optimal training can operate it without difficulty. A typical medical cyclotron is shown in Fig. 6-2. The cyclotrons from different manufacturers are listed in Table 6.1.

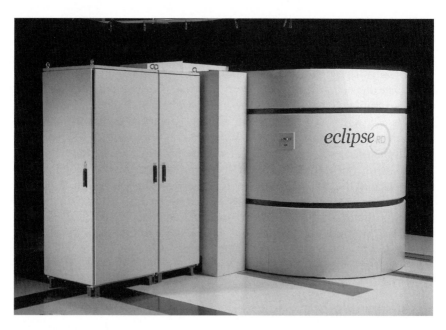

FIGURE 6-2. A commercial cyclotron, RDS ECLIPSE, developed and manufactured by CPS Innovations. (Courtesy of CPS Innovations, Knoxville, TN, USA.) The features of this cyclotron are given in Table 6.1.

Nuclear Reaction

When targets of stable elements are irradiated by placing them in the external beam or in the internal beam of accelerated particles at a given radius inside a cyclotron, the particles interact with the target nuclei and nuclear reactions take place. Depending on the kinetic energy, the incident particle may be completely absorbed, depositing all its energy, or may leave the

TABLE 6.1. Features of medical cyclotrons from different manufacturers.

Company	Model	Beam type	Particle energy (MeV)	Beam current (μA)	No of target positions	Simultaneous irradiation of targets
IBA	Cyclone 10/5	H$^-$/d$^-$	10/5	60/35	8	2
	Cyclone 18/9	H$^-$/d$^-$	18/9	80/35	8	2
CTI	RDS 111	H$^-$	11	50	8	2
	RDS ECLIPSE	H$^-$	11	50	8	2
GE Medical Solutions	PETtrace	H$^-$/d$^-$	16.5/8.5	75/60	6	2
EBCO	TR 30/15	H$^-$/d$^-$	30/15	400/150	8	2
	TR 19/9	H$^-$/d$^-$	19/9	150	8	2

nucleus after interaction with one or more nucleons, leaving part of its energy. Nuclear reactions involving very high-energy particles are called spallations, in which many nucleons are ejected from the nucleus by the direct interaction of the incident particle. In either case, an excited nucleus is formed, and the excitation energy is disposed of by the emission of protons and neutrons, provided it is energetically allowed. Particle emission is followed by a cascade of γ-ray emissions when the former is no longer energetically possible. Depending on the energy deposited, several nucleons may be emitted resulting in the production of different radionuclides. The larger the energy deposited, the more particles are emitted, and a variety of radionuclides are produced. A simple nuclear reaction induced by a proton p on a target $^{A}_{Z}X$ can be given by

$$^{A}_{Z}X(p,n)^{A}_{Z+1}Y$$

where n is the neutron emitted and $^{A}_{Z+1}Y$ is the radionuclide formed.

The target material for irradiation must be pure and preferably monoisotopic or at least enriched isotopically to avoid the production of extraneous radionuclides. Radionuclides are separated from the target material by appropriate chemical methods such as solvent extraction, precipitation, chromatography, ion exchange, and distillation. Cyclotron-produced radionuclides are typically neutron deficient and, therefore, decay by β^{+} emission or electron capture. Also, the radionuclides which are different from the target nuclides do not contain any stable (or "cold") atoms and are called *carrier-free*. Another term for these preparations is *no-carrier-added* (NCA), because no cold atoms have been intentionally added to the preparations.

Target and its Processing

Excessive heat is generated in the target during irradiation with charged particles at a beam current of 50 to 100 μA, and the temperature can rise, exceeding 1000°C. If proper precautions for heat dissipation are not taken, the target may be burned or melted. The most common method is to cool the probe to which the target is attached by using circulating water, helium gas, or other coolants. Also, the targets are designed in the form of a foil to maximize heat dissipation.

The common form of the target is the metallic foil, but metals melt at high temperature caused by high beam intensity of the particles. Other forms are oxides, carbonates, nitrates, etc., contained in the aluminum tubes, which are flattened after loading to maximize heat loss. The choice of aluminum is owing to its high melting point. In specific cases, high-pressure gas (e.g. ^{124}Xe for ^{123}I production) and liquid targets (e.g. $H_2^{18}O$ for ^{18}F production) are used. In the former case, the beam current is of the order of 10 to 40 μA and in the latter, it ranges between 10 and 25 μA.

Equation for Production of Radionuclides

The amount of activity produced by irradiation of a target material with a charged particle beam can be quantitated by

$$A = In\sigma(1 - e^{-\lambda t}) \tag{6.2}$$

where A = the activity in disintegration per second of the radionuclide produced.

I = intensity of irradiating particles (number of particles/cm^2·sec)

N = number of target atoms

σ = formation cross section (probability) of the radionuclide (cm^2); it is given in units of "barn," which is equal to 10^{-24} cm^2.

λ = decay constant of the radionuclide given by $0.693/t_{1/2}$ (sec^{-1}).

t = time of irradiation in seconds

Equation (6.2) indicates that the quantity of radionuclides increases with time of irradiation, intensity, and energy of the particles (related to σ) of the incident particle, and the amount of target material. The term ($1 - e^{-\lambda t}$) is called the saturation factor, which approaches to unity when t is 5 to 6 half-lives of the radionuclide in question. At that time, the yield of the radionuclide is maximum, and its rates of production and decay become equal, indicating that there is no gain in activity by further irradiation. For irradiation for five to six half-lives of the daughter, Eq. (6.2) then becomes

$$A = In\sigma \tag{6.3}$$

A graphic representation of Eqations (6.2) and (6.3) is shown in Figure 6-3.

The values of I are measured by various techniques, the description of which is beyond the scope of this book, but they are available from the cyclotron operators. The values of σ also have been determined for various nuclear reactions and are available in literature. The number of atoms N of the target is given by

$$N = \frac{W \times K}{A_w} \times 6.02 \times 10^{23} \tag{6.4}$$

where W is the weight of the target, A_w and K are the atomic weight and natural abundance of the target element, and 6.02×10^{23} is the Avogadro's number.

Note that 1 ampere is equal to 1 coulomb/sec, and 1 coulomb equals to 6.25×10^{18} protons, so in a cyclotron where protons or H$^-$ are accelerated, the beam intensity is conventionally expressed in $\mu A/cm^2$-hr. The yield of the radionuclide is then expressed in MBq or mCi per μAh.

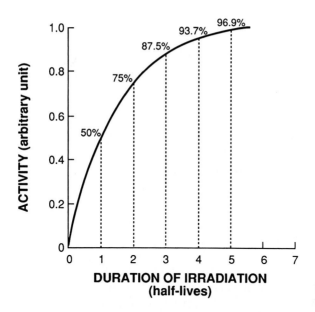

FIGURE 6-3. Production of radionuclides in a cyclotron. The amount of activity produced reaches a maximum (saturation) in 5 to 6 half-lives of the radionuclide.

Problem 6.1

Calculate the activity of ^{18}F produced when 1 gm of 70% enriched $H_2^{18}O$ is irradiated for 1 hr with a proton beam of $30\,\mu A/cm^2$ in a cyclotron. The half-life of ^{18}F is 110 min and the cross section for the ^{18}O (p,n) ^{18}F reaction is 300 millibarn (1 barn = 10^{-24} cm^2).

Answer:
Since 1 ampere is equal to 1 coulomb (C)/sec and 1 coulomb equals 6.25×10^{18} protons, the number of protons in $30\,\mu A/cm^2$ is

$$I = 30 \times 10^{-6} \times 6.25 \times 10^{18} = 1.875 \times 10^{14} \text{ protons}/(cm^2.sec)$$
$$\sigma = 0.3 \times 10^{-24} \text{ cm}^2$$

Effective molecular weight of enriched water is $0.3 \times 18 + 0.7 \times 20 = 19.4$.

$$N = \frac{0.7 \times 1}{19.4} \times 6.02 \times 10^{23} = 2.17 \times 10^{22} \text{ atoms} ^{18}O$$
$$\lambda = \frac{0.693}{110 \times 60} = 1.05 \times 10^{-4} \text{ sec}^{-1}$$
$$t = 1 \times 60 \times 60 = 3600 \text{ sec}$$

Using Eq. (6.1)

$$D(dps) = 1.875 \times 10^{14} \times 2.17 \times 10^{22} \times 0.3 \times 10^{-24}$$
$$\times [1 - \exp(-1.05 \times 10^{-4} \times 3600)]$$
$$= 1.22 \times 10^{12} \times 0.3148$$
$$= 3.84 \times 10^{11} dps(384\ GBq)$$
$$A = \frac{3.84 \times 10^{11}}{3.7 \times 10^{10}}$$
$$= 10.4\ Ci$$

Specific Activity

Specific activity of a sample is defined as the radioactivity per unit mass of a radionuclide or a labeled compound. If a 50 mg sample contains 100 mCi (370 MBq), then the specific activity of the sample is given as 100/50 = 2 mCi/mg or 74 MBq/mg. One should not confuse the specific activity with the concentration, which is given in mCi/ml or MBq/ml. The specific activity is at times expressed in units of mCi/mole (MBq/mole) or mCi/μmole (MBq/μmole).

The specific activity of a carrier-free radionuclide can be calculated by

$$\text{specific activity (mCi/mg)} = \frac{3.13 \times 10^9}{A \times t_{1/2}} \tag{6.5}$$

where   A = the mass number of the radionuclide
        $t_{1/2}$ = the half-life in hours of the radionuclide

The specific activity is an important parameter to consider in radio-labeling and *in vivo* biodistribution of tracers. Cold molecules in low-specific-activity radiopharmaceuticals compete with radioactive molecules and lower the uptake of the tracer in different organs. Similarly, low-specific-activity radionuclides yield poor radiolabeling.

Production of Positron-Emitting Radionuclides

Since only a limited number of short-lived radionuclides are useful for PET imaging, production of those in routine clinical use and a few with potential for future clinical use are described here. A few essential long-lived positron emitters are also included. The different characteristics of these radionuclides are summarized in Table 6.2.

TABLE 6.2. Production and characteristics of common positron emitters.

Nuclide	Physical half-life ($t_{1/2}$)	Mode of decay (%)	γ-ray energy (keV)	Abundance (%)	Common production method
$^{11}_{6}C$	20.4 min	β^+ (100)	511	200	$^{10}B(d,n)^{11}C$ $^{14}N(p,\alpha)^{11}C$
$^{13}_{7}N$	10 min	β^+ (100)	511	200	$^{12}C(d,n)^{13}N$ $^{16}O(p,\alpha)^{13}N$ $^{13}C(p,n)^{13}N$
$^{15}_{8}O$	2 min	β^+ (100)	511	200	$^{14}N(d,n)^{15}O$ $^{15}N(p,n)^{15}O$
$^{18}_{9}F$	110 min	β^+ (97) EC(3)	511	194	$^{18}O(p,n)^{18}F$
$^{68}_{31}Ga$	68 min	β^+ (89) EC(11)	511	178	$^{68}Ge—^{68}Ga$ generator $^{68}Zn(p,n)^{68}Ga$
$^{94m}_{43}Tc$	52 min	β^+ (70) EC(30)	511 871 1521 1868	140 94 4.5 5.7	$^{94}Mo(p,n)^{94m}Tc$
$^{124}_{53}I$	4.2 d	β^+ (23) EC(77)	511 603 1691	46 61 10.4	$^{124}Te(p,n)^{124}I$
$^{82}_{37}Rb$	75 s	β^+ (95) EC(5)	511 777	190 13.4	$^{98}Mo \xrightarrow{\text{spallation}} {}^{82}Sr$ $\downarrow 25.6 d$ ^{82}Rb

Fluorine-18

Fluorine-18 ($t_{1/2} = 110$ minutes) is commonly produced by the ^{18}O (p,n) ^{18}F reaction on a $H_2^{18}O$ target using 11 to 18 MeV protons in medical cyclotrons. $^{18}O\text{-}O_2$ gas target also has been used as the target for ^{18}F production, but has not received wide acceptance because of the low yield. $H_2^{18}O$ (85 to 99% enriched) is isotopically enriched target material in liquid form and is available from commercial vendors (e.g. Isotec, Inc., Miamisburg, OH, USA). A metal target holder (e.g. silver, titanium, nickel, copper, and stainless steel) with cavities of 0.1 to 4 cc volume is used to contain $H_2^{18}O$. Target design varies widely with the type and energy of the cyclotron. After irradiation, the target mixture is loaded on a column of carbonate ion exchange resin, and $H_2^{18}O$ is forced out of the column by neon gas and reused as the target. $^{18}F^-$ ion is recovered by eluting the column with potassium carbonate solution. Greater than curie (GBq) amount of ^{18}F-fluoride is easily produced in an 11 MeV cyclotron after bombardment for an hour. The NCA specific activity of ^{18}F-fluoride is in the order of about 1×10^4 Ci/mmol (3.7×10^5 GBq/mmol). ^{18}F-fluoride has been used for labeling deoxyglucose to produce ^{18}F-fluorodeoxyglucose (^{18}F-FDG), ^{18}F-fluorodopa, and a few other ^{18}F-labeled radiopharmaceuticals for PET imaging (discussed later).

Carbon-11

Carbon-11 has a half-life of 20.5 minutes and can be produced by $^{10}B(d,n)$ ^{11}C, $^{11}B(p,n)$ ^{11}C, and $^{14}N(p,\alpha)$ ^{11}C reactions in the cyclotron. In the first two reactions, B_2O_3 is the target and nitrogen gas in the third. Both ^{11}CO and $^{11}CO_2$ are produced in boron targets by using 10–12 MeV protons, which are then flushed out by neutral gases. Either ^{11}CO is oxidized to have all the gas in $^{11}CO_2$ form, or $^{11}CO_2$ is reduced to have all the gas in ^{11}CO form. Both ^{11}CO and $^{11}CO_2$ are commonly used as precursors in the preparation of various clinically useful compounds, such as ^{11}C-palmitate for myocardial metabolic imaging by PET.

The most common method of ^{11}C production is the $^{14}N(p,\alpha)$ ^{11}C reaction with 10–12 MeV protons. When the pure ^{14}N target is mixed with traces of oxygen, both ^{11}CO and $^{11}CO_2$ are produced. $^{11}CO_2$ is recovered by initially trapping $^{11}CO_2$ in a liquid nitrogen trap and later removing it by flushing with helium or heating the trap. The yield can be in curie (GBq) range with 99.9% purity.

The $^{14}N(p,\alpha)^{11}C$ reaction is carried out by bombardment of a mixture of N_2 and H_2 to give ^{11}C, which reacts with N_2 to produce ^{11}CN, followed by hydrolysis of ^{11}CN to give $^{11}CH_4$ (95% to 100% radiochemical yield). Carbon-11-methane is often allowed to react with NH_3 over platinum at 1000°C to give a 95% overall yield of $H^{11}CN$. Various biological molecules such as aliphatic amines, amino nitriles, and hydantoins have been labeled with ^{11}C using $H^{11}CN$ or $^{11}CH_4$ as a precursor. A frequently employed precursor for ^{11}C labeling is ^{11}C-methyl iodide, which is prepared by either converting ^{11}C-CO_2 to ^{11}C-methoxide followed by reaction with hydroiodic acid, or by a gas phase reaction where ^{11}C-CH_4 is reacted with iodine.

Nitrogen-13

Nitrogen-13 has a half-life of 10 minutes and is commonly used as NH_3. It is produced by the $^{12}C(d,n)^{13}N$ reaction by bombarding Al_4C_3 or methane with 6–7 MeV deuterons, or by the $^{16}O(p,\alpha)^{13}N$ or $^{13}C(p,n)^{13}N$ reaction. However, the $^{16}O(p,\alpha)^{13}N$ reaction is the most common method of ^{13}N production, and a target of pure water contained in a titanium holder is used for irradiation with 11–12 MeV protons. The major chemical species are nitrates, nitrites, ammonia, and hydroxylamine, of which the nitrate has the highest yield and is separated by the ion exchange method. The nitrates and nitrites are reduced to give $^{13}NH_3$ which is swept by helium into saline. $^{13}NH_3$ in the form of NH_4^+ ion is primarily used for myocardial perfusion imaging by PET. $^{13}NH_3$ is also used to label glutamine and asparagine for assessment of viability of tissues.

Oxygen-15

Oxygen-15 has a half-life of 2 minutes and is produced by the $^{14}N(d,n)^{15}O$ reaction by 8–10 MeV deuteron irradiation of gaseous nitrogen or by the $^{15}N(p,n)^{15}O$ reaction by 10–12 MeV proton bombardment of enriched ^{15}N

gas target contained in an aluminum alloy container. Pure ^{15}O gas is used for bolus and steady-state metabolic studies. ^{15}O$_2$ is passed over activated charcoal heated at 1000 degrees C to convert it to C^{15}O and C^{15}O$_2$, which are then used for labeling hemoglobins in clinical investigations of pulmonary and cardiac malfunctions. Oxygen-15 labeled water is obtained by heating a mixture of ^{15}O and hydrogen gas and is useful for cerebral and myocardial perfusion studies.

Iodine-124

Iodine-124 has a half-life of 4.2 days and is produced by the ^{124}Te (d,2n) ^{124}I or ^{124}Te (p,n) ^{124}I reaction using 10–18 MeV protons and a 96% enriched ^{124}Te target in the form of oxide. While it has the advantage of having a long half-life to produce suitable iodinated PET tracers, its low positron abundance (only 23%) and complex decay scheme involving high-energy photons cause difficulty in PET imaging.

Strontium-82

Rubidium-82 ($t_{1/2}$ = 75 seconds) is available from the ^{82}Sr–^{82}Rb generator (supplied by Bracco Diagnostics, Inc.). ^{82}Sr ($t_{1/2}$ = 25.6 days) is produced by the ^{85}Rb (p,4n) ^{82}Sr reaction using the high-energy proton beam on a ^{85}Rb target or by the spallation reaction of ^{99}Mo target with very high-energy protons, the latter being the preferred reaction. The ^{82}Sr radionuclide is separated from the target by the ion-exchange method. The purified ^{82}Sr in amounts of 90 mCi to 150 mCi (3.33 GBq to 5.55 GBq) is loaded on a stannic oxide column in the generator. ^{82}Rb is eluted as chloride with 0.9% sodium chloride solution from the ^{82}Sr–^{82}Rb generator by using an infusion pump. (See Chapter 11.). The major impurities in the ^{82}Sr sample are ^{85}Sr ($t_{1/2}$ = 65 d) and ^{83}Sr ($t_{1/2}$ = 32 hours). While ^{85}Sr contamination can be as much as five times the ^{82}Sr activity in the range of 400 mCi to 700 mCi (14.8 GBq to 25.9 GBq) when produced using the ^{98}Mo target, it is significantly less when the ^{85}Rb target is used. However, ^{83}Sr decays to a negligible quantity by the time ^{82}Sr is loaded on the generator column.

Technetium-94m

Technetium-94m ($t_{1/2}$ = 52 minutes) is produced by the ^{94}Mo (p,n) ^{94m}Tc reaction using an enriched ^{94}Mo target and 11 to 12 MeV protons. ^{94m}Tc is separated from ^{94}Mo by steam distillation. It is an attractive positron emitter since it can be substituted for ^{99m}Tc in many SPECT radiopharmaceuticals for use in PET imaging.

Germanium-68

Germanium-68 (t$_{1/2}$ = 270.8 days) is mainly used as a sealed source for transmission scan and quality control studies in PET imaging. It is produced by the ^{66}Zn(α,2n)^{68}Ge reaction, or the 40-MeV proton bombardment of a gallium target, or the spallation reactions in a molybdenum target with high-energy protons. It decays by electron capture and remains in equilibrium with ^{68}Ga ($t_{1/2}$ = 68 minutes). It is also used in the ^{68}Ge-^{68}Ga generator to provide easy supply of ^{68}Ga.

Questions

1. Describe the principles of the operation of a cyclotron.
2. What is the major advantage of a negative ion cyclotron over a positive ion cyclotron?
3. Why is the higher vacuum required in a negative ion cyclotron than in a positive ion cyclotron?
4. Describe the production of the following radionuclides in a cyclotron. (A) ^{13}N, (B) ^{11}C, (C) ^{18}F, and (D) ^{15}O.
5. Radionuclides produced in a cyclotron are typically carrier-free or NCA. True _____; False _____.
6. Calculate the activity of ^{18}F when 700 mg of 85% enriched $H_2^{18}O$ is irradiated for 1 hour with a proton beam of $20\,\mu A/cm^2$ in a cyclotron. The half-life of ^{18}F is 110 minutes and the cross section for the ^{18}O (p,n) ^{18}F reaction is 200 millibarn (1 barn = $10^{-24}\,cm^2$).
7. In producing a radionuclide with $t_{1/2}$ = 3 hours in a cyclotron, what is the duration of irradiation after which there is no more gain in additional activity?
8. What are the chemical forms of ^{18}F that are obtained at the end of bombardment to be used for further chemical synthesis?
9. The specific activity of a radioactive sample decreases with the increasing cold atoms. True _____; False _____.
10. Calculate the specific activity of a carrier-free ^{18}F sample.

Suggested Reading

1. Friedlander G, Kennedy JW, Miller JM. *Nuclear and Radiochemistry.* 3rd ed. New York: Wiley. 1981.
2. McCarthy TJ, Welch MJ. The state of positron emitting radionuclide production in 1997. *Semin Nucl Med.* 1998;XXVII:235.
3. Saha GB, MacIntyre WJ, Go RT. Cyclotrons and positron emission tomography for clinical imaging. *Semin Nucl Med.* 1992;22:150.
4. Saha GB. *Fundamentals of Nuclear Pharmacy.* 5th ed. New York: Springer-Verlag; 2004.
5. Silvester DJ, Waters SL. Radionuclide production. In: Sodd VJ, Allen DR, Hoogland DR, Ice RD, eds. *Radiopharmaceuticals II.* New York: Society of Nuclear Medicine; 1979:727.

7
Synthesis of PET Radiopharmaceuticals

PET radiopharmaceuticals are uniquely different from SPECT radiopharmaceuticals in that the former have radionuclides that are positron emitters and the majority of them have short physical half-lives. The most common PET radionuclides are ^{11}C, ^{15}O, ^{13}N, ^{18}F, and ^{82}Rb, which are short-lived (See Table 6.2) and put limitations on the synthesis time for PET radiopharmaceuticals and their clinical use. The attractive advantage of PET radiopharmaceuticals, however, is that the ligands used in radiopharmaceuticals are common analogs of biological molecules, and therefore, often depict a true representation of biological processes after in vivo administration. For example, ^{18}F-fluorodeoxyglucose (FDG) is an analog of glucose used for cellular metabolism and $H_2{}^{15}O$ for cerebral perfusion.

Many radiopharmaceuticals have been used for PET imaging; however, only a few are routinely utilized for clinical purposes. Almost all of them are labeled with one of the four common positron emitters: ^{11}C, ^{13}N, ^{15}O, and ^{18}F. Of the four, ^{18}F is preferred most, since it has a relatively longer half-life ($t_{1/2} = 110$ min) that allows its supply to remote places. In all cases, a suitable synthesis method is adopted to provide a stable product with good labeling yield, high specific activity, high purity, and most importantly, high in vivo tissue selectivity. For example, ^{82}Rb is used as a PET radiotracer in the form of ^{82}Rb-RbCl that is available from the ^{82}Sr-^{82}Rb generator. The following is a description of the syntheses of the common clinically used PET radiopharmaceuticals and a few with potential for future use.

PET Radiopharmaceuticals

^{18}F-Sodium Fluoride

Fluorine-18 ($t_{1/2} = 110$ minutes) is produced by irradiation of ^{18}O-water with 10 to 18 MeV protons in a cyclotron and recovered as ^{18}F-sodium fluoride by passing the irradiated water target mixture through a carbonate type anion exchange resin column. The water passes through, whereas $^{18}F^-$ is retained on the column, which is recovered by elution with potassium carbonate solution. Its pH should be between 4.5 to 8.0. While ^{18}F-sodium fluoride is most commonly used for the synthesis of ^{18}F-fluorodeoxyglucose, it is also used for other ^{18}F-labeled PET radiopharmaceuticals. The U.S. FDA has approved it for bone scintigraphy, since it localizes in bone by exchanging with PO_4^- ion in the hydroxyapatite crystal.

^{18}F-Fluorodeoxyglucose (FDG)

^{18}F-2-fluoro-2-deoxyglucose (2-FDG) is normally produced in places where a cyclotron is locally available. Its molecular formula is $C_8H_{11}{}^{18}FO_5$ with molecular weight of 181.3 daltons. ^{18}F-2-FDG can be produced by electrophilic substitution with ^{18}F-fluorine gas or nucleophilic displacement with ^{18}F-fluoride ions. The radiochemical yield is low with the electrophilic substitution, so the nucleophilic displacement reaction has become the method of choice for ^{18}F-FDG synthesis. Deoxyglucose is labeled with ^{18}F by nucleophilic displacement reaction of an acetylated sugar derivative followed by hydrolysis (Hamacher et al., 1986). In nucleophilic substitution, a fluoride ion reacts to fluorinate the sugar derivative. A solution of 1,3,4,6-tetra-O-acetyl-2-O-trifluoromethane-sulfonyl-β-D-mannopyranose in anhydrous acetonitrile is added to a dry residue of ^{18}F-fluoride containing aminopolyether (Kryptofix 2.2.2) and potassium carbonate (Figure 7-1). Kryptofix 2.2.2 is used as a catalyst to enhance the reactivity of the fluoride ions. The mixture is heated under reflux for about 5 minutes. The solution is then passed through a C-18 Sep-Pak column, and acetylated carbohydrates are eluted with tetrahydrofuran (THF), which are then

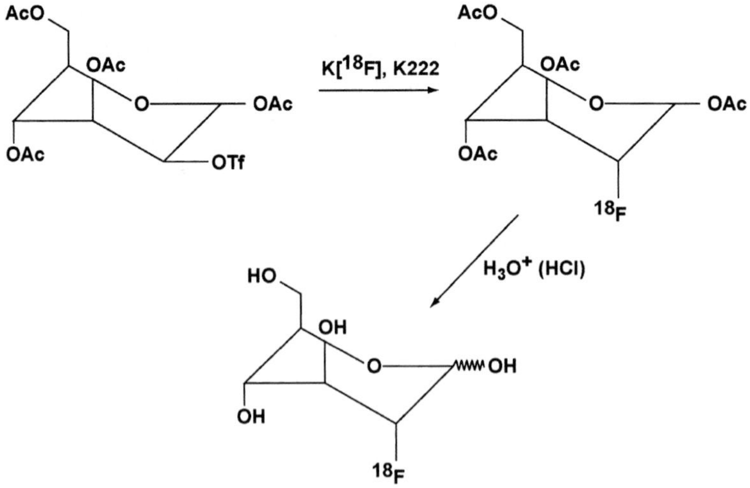

FIGURE 7-1. Schematic synthesis of ^{18}F-2-Fluoro-2-deoxyglucose (FDG). (Reprinted with the permission of the Cleveland Clinic Foundation.)

hydrolyzed by refluxing in hydrochloric acid at 130°C for 15 minutes. ^{18}F-2-fluoro-2-deoxyglucose (2-FDG) is obtained by passing the hydrolysate through a C-18 Sep-Pak column. The yield can be as high as 60%, and the preparation time is approximately 50 minutes. The final solution is filtered through a $0.22 \mu m$ filter and diluted with saline, as needed. It should have a pH of 7.0.

Since Kryptofix 2.2.2 is toxic causing apnea and convulsions, modifications have been made to substitute it with tetrabutylammonium hydroxide or bicarbonate, which have been adopted by many commercial vendors. Also, in some other methods, the C-18 Sep-Pak column separation has been eliminated so as to carry out the acidic hydrolysis in the same vessel. In methods where Kryptofix 2.2.2 is still used, several Sep-Pak columns are used to separate Kryptofix 2.2.2 and reduce it to practically a negligible quantity.

[18]F-2-FDG is used primarily for the study of metabolism in the brain and heart, and for the detection of epilepsy and various tumors. In metabolism, ^{18}F-2-FDG is phosphorylated by hexokinase to 2-FDG-6-phosphate which is not metabolized further. It should be noted that 3-fluoro-deoxyglucose (3-FDG) is not phosphorylated and hence is not trapped and essentially eliminated rapidly from the cell. This is why 3-FDG is not used for metabolic studies.

6-^{18}F-L-Fluorodopa

Like ^{18}F-2-FDG, 6-^{18}F-L-fluorodopa is also produced in places where a cyclotron is available locally. There are several methods of synthesizing 6-^{18}F-fluoro-3,4-dihydroxyphenylalanine (6-^{18}F-L-fluorodopa), of which the method of fluorodemetallation using electrophilic fluorinating agents is most widely used. Electrophilic reactions involve the reaction of fluorine in the form of F^+ with other molecules. Only the L-isomer of dopa is important, because the enzymes that convert dopa to dopamine, which is targeted by the radiopharmaceutical, are selective for this isomer. Initially, a suitably protected organomercury precursor (N-[trifluoroacetyl]-3,4-dimethoxy-6-trifluoroacetoxymercuriophenylalanine ethyl ester) of dopa is prepared. [^{18}F]-labeled acetylhypofluorite prepared in the gas phase is then allowed to react with the mercury precursor in chloroform or acetonitrile at room temperature. Other precursors using metals such as tin, silicon, selenium and germanium have been reported. Acid hydrolysis with 47% HBr provides a relatively high yield (10–12%) of 6-^{18}F-L-fluorodopa (Luxen et al., 1987), compared to other available methods. Substitution at position 6 is most desirable, because this does not alter the behavior of dopa, whereas substitutions at 2 and 5 do. It is sterilized by filtering through a $0.22 \mu m$ membrane filter, and is supplied at pH between 4.0 and 5.0. Normally EDTA and ascorbic acid are added to the final preparation for stability. The molecular structure of 6-^{18}F-L-fluorodopa is shown in

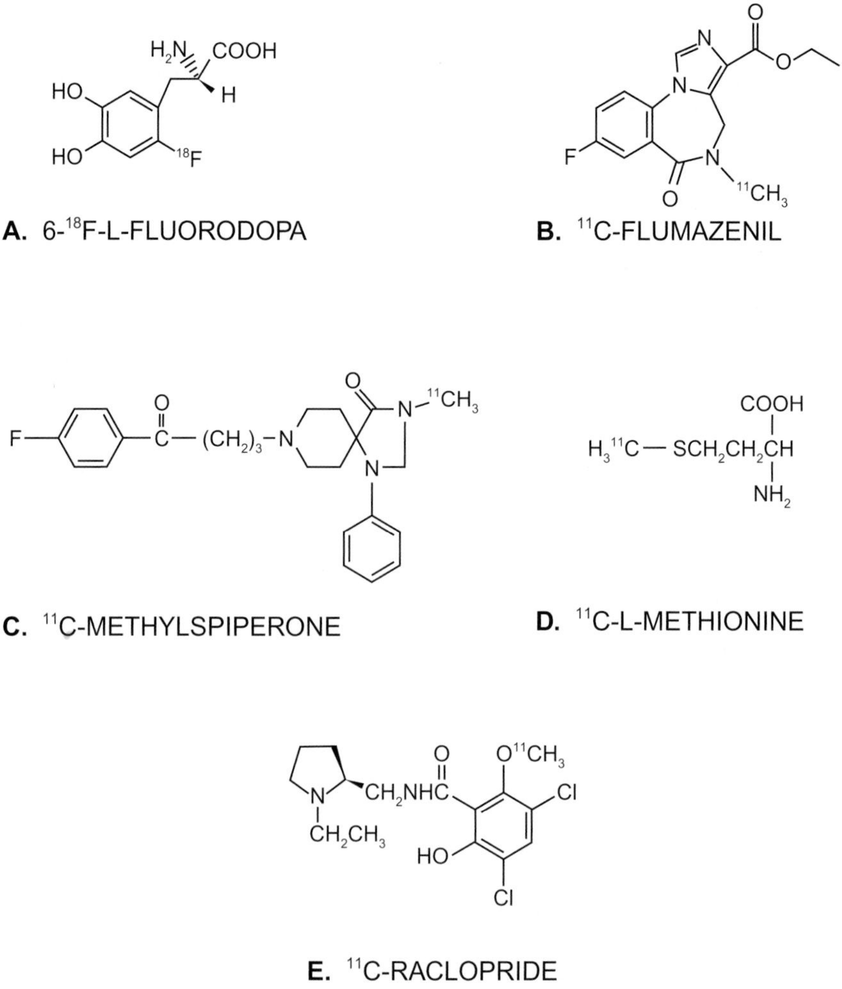

A. 6-¹⁸F-L-FLUORODOPA

B. ¹¹C-FLUMAZENIL

C. ¹¹C-METHYLSPIPERONE

D. ¹¹C-L-METHIONINE

E. ¹¹C-RACLOPRIDE

FIGURE 7-2. Molecular structures of (A) 6-^{18}F-L-fluorodopa, (B) ^{11}C-flumazenil, (C) ^{11}C-methylspiperone, (D) ^{11}C-L-methionine, (E) ^{11}C-raclopride. (Reprinted with the permission of the Cleveland Clinic Foundation.)

Figure 7-2A. 6-^{18}F-L-fluorodopa is used for the assessment of the presynaptic dopaminergic function in the brain.

^{18}F-Fluorothymidine (FLT)

^{18}F-fluorothymidine (FLT) is prepared by nucleophilic reaction between ^{18}F-sodium fluoride and a precursor, 2,3′-anhydro-5′-0-benzoyl-2′-deoxythymidine, which is prepared by standard organic synthesis (Machulla et al., 2000). ^{18}F-sodium fluoride is added to a mixture of Kryptofix 2.2.2

and potassium carbonate in acetonitrile, and the mixture is dried to a residue by heating at 120°C for 5 minutes. The precursor in dimethyl sulfoxide (DMSO) is added to the dried residue and heated at 160°C for 10 minutes. Hydrolysis of the 5'-0-protecting group is performed with sodium hydroxide. ^{18}F-FLT is isolated by passing through alumina Sep-Pak and further purified by using HPLC. The overall yield is about 45% and the radiochemical purity is more than 95%. The synthesis time is about 60 minutes.

Since thymidine is incorporated into DNA and provides a measure of cell proliferation, ^{18}F-FLT is commonly used for in vivo diagnosis and characterization of tumors in humans.

^{15}O-Water

^{15}O-oxygen ($t_{1/2}$ = 2 minutes) is produced in the cyclotron by the ^{15}N(p, n)^{15}O reaction, or the ^{14}N(d, n)^{15}O reaction, and the irradiated gas is transferred to a [^{15}O] water generator in which ^{15}O is mixed with hydrogen and passed over a palladium/charcoal catalyst at 170°C (Meyer et al., 1986; Welch and Kilbourn, 1985). The $H_2^{15}O$ vapor is trapped in saline, and the saline solution is filtered through a 0.22μm membrane filter. The sample is then passed through a radiation detector for radioassay and ultimately injected on-line into a patient in a very short time.

$H_2^{15}O$ is commonly used for myocardial and cerebral perfusion studies.

n-^{15}O-Butanol

n-^{15}O-butanol is prepared by the reaction of ^{15}O-oxygen, produced by the ^{15}N(p, n)^{15}O reaction, with tri-n-butyl borane loaded onto an alumina Sep-Pak cartridge (Kabalka et al., 1985). Carrier oxygen at a concentration of about 0.5% is added to the ^{15}N target in order to recover ^{15}O. After the reaction, n-^{15}O-butanol is eluted from the cartridge with water. It is further purified by passing through C-18 Sep-Pak and eluting with ethanol-water.

n-^{15}O-butanol is used for blood flow measurement in the brain and other organs. It is a better perfusion agent than ^{15}O-water, because its partition coefficient is nearly 1.0 compared to 0.9 for water.

^{13}N-Ammonia

Nitrogen-13-labeled ammonia ($t_{1/2}$ = 10 minutes) is produced by reduction of ^{13}N-labeled nitrates and nitrites that are produced by proton irradiation of water in a cyclotron. The reduction is carried out with titanium chloride in alkaline medium. ^{13}N-NH$_3$ is then distilled and finally trapped in acidic saline solution. Wieland et al. (1991) have used a pressurized target of aqueous ethanol, in which ethanol acts as a hydroxyl free radical scavenger to improve the yield of ^{13}N-NH$_3$. The mixture is passed through an anion-exchange resin to remove all anion impurities. It is filtered through a 0.22μm membrane filter and its pH should be between 4.5 and 7.5. The US FDA has approved it for measurement of myocardial and cerebral perfusion.

^{11}C-Sodium Acetate

^{11}C-sodium acetate is produced by the reaction of the Grignard reagent, methylmagnesium bromide in diethyl ether, with cyclotron-produced ^{11}C-carbon dioxide at ambient temperature. After reaction, the product is hydrolyzed with water or aqueous acid, followed by further purification using the solvent extraction or ion exchange method. The solution is filtered through a 0.22μm membrane filter. ^{11}C-acetate has been found to be stable at pH between 4.5 and 8.5 for up to 2 hours at room temperature. The overall yield is about 75%. It is used for the measurement of oxygen consumption (oxidative metabolism) in the heart, since acetyl CoA synthetase converts ^{11}C-acetate to acetyl coenzyme A after myocardial uptake, which is metabolized to ^{11}C-CO$_2$ in the tricarboxylic acid cycle.

^{11}C-Flumazenil

^{11}C-flumazenil is commonly labeled at the N-methyl position by N-methylation with ^{11}C-iodomethane, which is prepared from ^{11}C-CO$_2$, and using the freshly prepared Grignard reagent, methylmagnesium bromide. The specific activity is very important for this product and therefore is analyzed by HPLC to give an optimum value between 0.5 and 2 Ci/μmol (18.5 to 74 GBq/μmol). It remains stable for up to 3 hours at room temperature at pH 7.0. The molecular structure of ^{11}C-fumazenil is shown in Figure 7-2B.

Since it is a benzodiazepine receptor ligand, ^{11}C-flumazenil is primarily used for the neuroreceptor characterization in humans.

^{11}C-Methylspiperone (MSP)

^{11}C-methylspiperone (MSP) is prepared by N-methylation of commercially available spiperone with ^{11}C-methyl iodide in the presence of Grignard reagent, methylmagnesium bromide, using different solvents and bases (Mazière et al., 1992). Since spiperones are sensitive to bases and to radiolysis at high level of activity, the yield of ^{11}C-MSP has been variable for different investigators. Cold spiperone present in the preparation reduces its specific activity and should be controlled. Specific activity should be around 10 to 50 GBq/mol (270 to 1350 mCi/mol). High specific activity ^{11}C-MSP undergoes autodecomposition in saline due to radiation, and a hydroxyl radical scavenger (e.g. ethanol) is added to prevent it. The final preparation is filtered through a 0.22μm membrane filter and its pH is adjusted to 7 ± 1 with a suitable buffer. The molecular structure of ^{11}C-methylspiperone is shown in Figure 7-2C.

^{11}C-methylspiperone is primarily used to determine the dopamine-2 receptor density in patients with neurological disorders, because of its high affinity for D-2 receptors in the brain.

^{11}C-L-Methionine

^{11}C-L-methionine has ^{11}C at its methyl position and has 2 forms: L-[1-^{11}C] methionine and L-[S-methyl-^{11}C] methionine. The former is obtained by the reaction between ^{11}C-CO_2 precursor and carbanion produced by a strong base added to the respective isonitrile, followed by hydrolysis with an acid. The latter is obtained by alkylation of the sulfide anion of L-homocysteine with ^{11}C-iodomethane. The product is purified by HPLC yielding a purity of >98% and further filtered through a $0.22\,\mu m$ membrane filter. The pH should be between 6.0 and 8.0 and it is stable for 2 hours at room temperature. The molecular structure of ^{11}C-L-methionine is shown in Figure 7-2D.

This compound is used for the detection of different types of malignancies, reflecting the amino acid utilization (transport, protein synthesis, transmethylation, etc.).

^{11}C-Raclopride

Raclopride is labeled with ^{11}C either by N-ethylation with [1-^{11}C] iodoethane or by O-methylation with [^{11}C] iodomethane, although the latter is more suitable for routine synthesis. Both ^{11}C-labeled iodoethane and iodomethane are prepared from ^{11}C-CO_2. The product is purified by HPLC giving a purity of greater than 98%. The specific activity should be in the range of 0.5 to $2\,Ci/\mu mol$ (18.5 to $74\,GBq/\mu mol$). The product at pH between 4.5 and 8.5 remains stable for more than 1 hr at room temperature. The molecular structure of ^{11}C-raclopride is shown in Figure 7-2E.

^{11}C-raclopride is primarily used to detect various neurological and psychiatric disorders, such as Parkinson's disease, schizophrenia, etc.

^{82}Rb-Rubidium Chloride

^{82}Rb-rubidium chloride is available from the ^{82}Sr-^{82}Rb generator, which is manufactured and supplied monthly by Bracco Diagnostics. The activity in the column is typically 90 to 150 mCi (3.33 to 5.55 GBq) ^{82}Sr at calibration time. ^{82}Rb is eluted with saline and must be checked for ^{82}Sr and ^{85}Sr breakthrough daily before the start of its use for patient studies. The allowable limit for ^{82}Sr is $0.02\,\mu Ci/mCi$ or 0.02 kBq/MBq of ^{82}Rb and the limit for ^{85}Sr is $0.2\,\mu Ci/mCi$ or 0.2 kBq/MBq of ^{82}Rb. Since ^{82}Rb has a short half-life of 75 seconds, it is administered to the patient by an infusion pump (see Chapter 11). The administered activity is the integrated activity infused at a certain flow rate for a period of time set by the operator, which is provided on the printout by a printer.

^{82}Rb is approved by the FDA for myocardial perfusion imaging to delineate ischemia from infarction.

Automated Synthesis Devices

Conventional manual methods of synthesis of radiopharmaceuticals using a high level of radioactivity are likely to subject the persons involved in the synthesis to high radiation exposure. This is particularly true with short-lived positron emitters such as ^{11}C, ^{13}N, ^{15}O, and ^{18}F, because the quantity of these radionuclides handled in the synthesis is very high. To minimize the level of exposure, automated modules have been devised for the synthesis of PET radiopharmaceuticals.

The automated synthesis device, often called the *black box*, is a unit controlled by microprocessors and software programs to carry out the sequential physical and chemical steps to accomplish the entire synthesis of a radiolabeled product. The unit consists of templates or vials pre-filled with required chemicals attached to the apparatus via tubings that are connected to solenoid values to switch on and off as needed. Most black boxes are small enough to be placed in a space of $20 \times 20 \times 20$ inches, and are capable of self-cleaning. In some units, disposable cassettes are employed so that new cassettes can be used for each new synthesis. Various parameters for synthesis such as time, pressure, volume and other requisites are all controlled by a remote computer. The unit has a graphic display showing the status of the on-going process. After the synthesis, a report with the date, start and end time of the radiosynthesis, and the calculated yield is printed out. Technologists can operate these units very easily. Automated synthesis modules for ^{18}F-FDG, ^{13}N-NH$_3$, ^{11}C-CH$_3$I, ^{11}C-HCN, ^{11}C-acetate, and a few other PET tracers are commercially available. A schematic diagram of a black box for ^{18}F-FDG synthesis is shown in Figure 7-3. An automated FDG synthesis module marketed by CTI Molecular Imaging, PET NET is shown in Figure 7-4. Other vendors include GE Medical Systems (Tracerlab), Siemens, Bioscan, EBCO and Sumitomo.

Quality Control of PET Radiopharmaceuticals

As with conventional drugs, PET radiopharmaceuticals must be tested for chemical purity, radionuclidic purity, radiochemical purity, pH, isotonicity, sterility, apyrogenicity, and toxicity prior to administration to humans. Because PET radiopharmaceuticals are short-lived, many tests cannot be performed in a short time just before administration. In these cases, quality control tests are performed on the products using "dry runs" without administration to patients and the method of production is validated. At

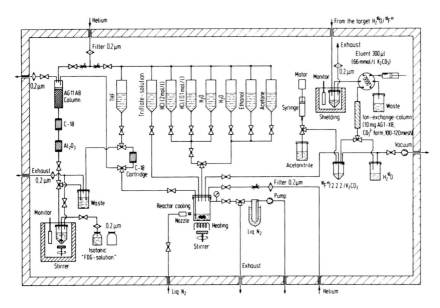

FIGURE 7-3. A schematic block diagram showing different components in the ^{18}F-FDG synthesis box. (Reproduced with kind permission of Kluwer Academic Publishers from Crouzel C, et al. Radiochemistry automation PET. In: Stöcklin G, Pike VW, eds. *Radiopharmaceuticals for Positron Emission Tomography*. Dordrecht, The Netherlands, Kluwer Academic; 1993; p. 64. Fig. 9.)

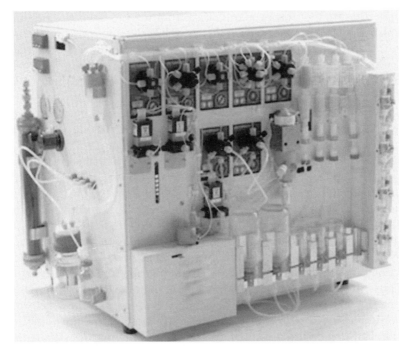

FIGURE 7-4. An automated ^{18}F-FDG synthesis box, Explora-FDG4, manufactured by CTI Molecular Imaging, PET NET. (Courtesy of CPS Innovations, Knoxville, TN, USA.)

times, tests for very short-lived PET tracers may need to be performed on an "after-the-fact" basis.

The quality control tests can be divided into two categories: physicochemical tests and biological tests. Refer to Saha (2004) for detailed description of these methods. These tests are briefly outlined below.

Physicochemical Tests

Physicochemical tests include the tests for the physical and chemical parameters of a PET radiopharmaceutical, namely physical appearance, isotonicity, pH, radionuclidic purity, chemical purity, and radiochemical purity.

Physical Appearance: Physical appearance relates to the color, clarity or turbidity of a PET radiopharmaceutical and should be checked by visual inspection of the sample.

pH: The pH of a PET radiopharmaceutical for human administration should be ideally 7.4, but both slightly acidic and basic pH values are tolerated due to the buffer capacity of the blood. The pH can be adjusted by adding appropriate buffer to the solution.

Isotonicity: Isotonicity is the ionic strength of a solution, which is mainly adjusted by adding appropriate electrolytes. Normally PET radiopharmaceuticals have appropriate isotonicity for human administration.

Radionuclidic Purity: The radionuclidic purity of a radiopharmaceutical is the fraction of total activity in the form of the desired radionuclide in the sample. These impurities primarily arise from the radionuclides produced by various nuclear reactions in a target as well as the impurities in the target material. Using a multichannel spectrometer, one can determine the level of impurities in a sample of a positron-emitting radionuclide produced by a specific nuclear reaction in a cyclotron. Using highly pure target material and appropriate chemical separation techniques, the radionuclidic purity can be minimized to an acceptable level. Short-lived radionuclides can be allowed to decay to have a pure relatively long-lived radionuclide in question. Even though the impurities in the routine preparations of PET radionuclides do not vary significantly from batch to batch, periodic checkup is recommended to validate the integrity of the method of production. The radionuclidic impurities must be established in ^{11}C, ^{13}N, ^{15}O, and ^{18}F radionuclides, prior to their use in the synthesis of radiolabeled compounds.

Chemical Purity: Chemical purity is the fraction of a radiopharmaceutical in the form of the desired chemical molecule whether all of it is radiolabeled or not. The presence of extraneous stable atoms may cause adverse reactions and is not desirable in a PET radiopharmaceutical. These impurities arise from the incomplete synthesis, addition of extraneous ingredients during the synthesis, and so on. Chemical methods such as the spectrophotometric method, ion exchange, solvent extractions, chromatography, etc. are applied to measure the level of these chemical impurities. Again, these tests can be performed a priori in many dry runs and thus the level of chemical impurities can be established, prior to human administration.

Radiochemical Purity: The radiochemical purity of a radiopharmaceutical is defined as the fraction of the total activity in the desired chemical form in the sample. These impurities arise from incomplete labeling, breakdown of the labeled products over time due to instability, and introduction of extraneous labeled ingredients during synthesis. These impurities cause altered in vivo biodistribution after administration, resulting in an unnecessary radiation dose to the patient. For these reasons, the United States Pharmacopea (USP) and the United States Food and Drug Administration have set limits on the impurities in various radiopharmaceuticals, and these limits must not be exceeded in clinical operations.

Since most PET radiopharmaceuticals are produced on site daily, the radiochemical purity must be checked for each batch. For very short-lived radionuclides, however, the methodology must be validated beforehand by carrying out many dry runs so that the radiochemical purity of the product remains within the limit set for human administration.

Various analytical methods are employed to establish the radiochemical purity of PET radiopharmaceuticals. The most common method is high-performance liquid chromatography (HPLC), which gives separation of components with high resolution. The general principle of HPLC involves forcing a sample at high pressure through a column of special packing material by an electric pump, whereby various components pass out of the column at different rates depending on their molecular weights. The fractions are collected at different times. The different components can then be identified and quantitated either by counting the radioactivity in each fraction with a counter, or by measuring their absorbance with an ultraviolet (UV) monitor.

Another common method of determining the radiochemical purity is the thin layer chromatography (TLC). In this method, a drop of the radiopharmaceutical sample is spotted on a solid phase paper strip (e.g., silica gel, Whatman) and then the paper is placed vertically in a jar containing a small amount of an appropriate solvent, taking care that the spotted area remains above the solvent. The solvent flows along the paper strip, and different components of the sample will flow at different rates along the strip depending on their solubility in the solvent. The ratio of the distance traveled by a component to the distance traveled by the solvent front is called the R_f value. When the solvent front reaches the top of the strip, the strip is removed and scanned for the distribution of components along the strip. Alternatively, the strip is cut into several segments (e.g., 10 segments), and the activity in each segment is measured by a counter. From the counts of the segments, the radiochemical purity can be calculated.

Biological Tests

Biological tests include sterility testing, pyrogen testing, and toxicity testing.

Sterility: Sterility indicates the absence of any viable bacteria or microorganisms in a radiopharmaceutical preparation. All radiopharmaceuticals must be sterile prior to administration to humans, and it is normally accomplished by filtering the product through a $0.22\,\mu m$ membrane filter, or heating the sample to 120°C for 20 minutes at a pressure of 18 pounds per square inch. PET radiopharmaceuticals are normally sterilized by filtration because of their short half-life.

Sterility tests are normally performed by incubating the sample with fluid thioglycollate medium at 30° to 35°C for 14 days or with soybean-casein digest medium at 20° to 25°C for 14 days. The sample volume should be as large as that for human dosage. If bacterial growth is observed in either test, the preparation is considered asterile. For PET radiopharmaceuticals, these tests are performed "after the fact" because of their short half-life.

Pyrogenicity: Pyrogens are polysaccharides or proteins produced by the metabolism of microorganisms, and upon administration, cause undue symptoms such as fever, flushing, chill, sweating, malaise, etc. These symptoms typically set in 30 minutes to 2 hours after administration and are rarely fatal. There are no specific methods of making a preparation pyrogen-free, and the only way to avoid pyrogens is to strictly follow the method of preparation employing meticulous aseptic technique so that microbes are not introduced into the sample.

Tests for pyrogens include a rabbit test, in which rabbits are administered with the radiopharmaceutical and their rectal temperatures are monitored. From the rise in temperature in the rabbits, pyrogenicity of a sample is determined. However, a simpler and quicker method is the so-called *limsulus amebocyte lysate* (LAL) test. In this test, the lysate of amebocytes from the blood of the horseshoe crab (*limulus polyphemus*) is mixed with the sample and incubated at 37°C. An opaque gel is formed within 15 to 60 minutes depending on the concentration of pyrogens. For PET radiopharmaceuticals, these tests are performed "after the fact".

Toxicity: The toxicity of a radiopharmaceutical causes alteration in the histology or physiologic functions of an organ or even death of a species after in vivo administration. It is commonly characterized by $LD_{50/60}$, which is defined as the quantity of a sample that kills 50% of the species within 60 days after administration. It must be established at least in two species before human administration, and the dosage to the humans is decided by a large safety factor. Toxicity arises from the pharmaceutical part and most PET radiopharmaceuticals are not toxic for human administration.

USP Specifications for Routine PET Radiopharmaceuticals

^{18}F-fluorodeoxyglucose

Appearance:	Clear
pH:	4.5 to 7.5

Specific Activity:	Not less than 1 Ci (37 GBq)/μmol
Radionuclidic Purity:	Not less than 99.5% should correspond to 511 keV, 1.022 MeV or Compton scatter peaks of ^{18}F.
Chemical Purity:	Major impurities are Kryptofix 2.2.2 and 2-chloro-2-deoxy-D-glucose, which are determined by TLC. Kryptofix 2.2.2 should not exceed 50 μg/ml of the sample volume, and 2-chloro-2-deoxy-D-glucose should not exceed 1 mg per total volume of the batch produced.
Radiochemical Purity:	It is determined by TLC using activated silica gel as the solid phase and a mixture of acetonitrile and water (95:5) as the solvent. The R_f value of ^{18}F-FDG is 0.4. The radiochemical purity should be more than 90%.

6-^{18}F-L-Fluorodopa

Appearance:	Clear
pH:	6 to 7
Specific Activity:	Not less than 100 mCi (3.7 GBq)/mmol
Radionuclidic Purity:	Not less than 99.5% correspond to 511 keV, 1.022 MeV or Compton scatter peaks of ^{18}F, with no individual impurity present more than 0.1%.
Chemical Purity:	Since the most common method of production utilizes organo mercury precursor, mercury is the major toxic impurity. It is determined by atomic absorption spectrometry and its USP limit is 0.5 μg/ml of L-dopa solution.
Radiochemical Purity:	It is determined by the HPLC method or ion pair chromatography. The USP limit is 95% of the total radioactivity in the form of 6-^{18}F-L-fluorodopa.

^{13}N-Ammonia

Appearance:	Clear
pH:	4.5 to 7.5
Specific Activity:	no carrier added
Radionuclidic Purity:	Not less than 99.5% should correspond to 511 keV, 1.022 MeV and Compton scatter of ^{13}N.
Chemical Purity:	Aluminum and titanium are the common impurities, determined by colorimetric methods. The USP limit of Al^{3+} is 10 μg/ml of the solution.
Radiochemical Purity:	It is determined by the HPLC method. The radiochemical yield should be greater than 95%.

Questions

1. Describe in detail the method of ^{18}F-FDG synthesis.
2. Describe the method of synthesis of: (a) 6-^{18}F-L-Fluorodopa; (b) ^{18}F-fluorothymidine; (c) ^{11}C-L-methionine.
3. What is the difference between the nucleophilic and electrophilic reaction?
4. What are the clinical uses of ^{18}F-FDG, ^{18}F-FLT, 6-^{18}F-L-Fluorodopa, ^{15}O-Water, ^{13}N-Ammonia, ^{11}C-Sodium acetate, and ^{11}C-Methylspiperone.
5. Describe the operational principles of an automated synthesis box.
6. Define (a) radionuclide purity, (b) radiochemical purity, (c) chemical purity of a radiopharmaceutical.
7. Describe the method of determining the radiochemical purity of a ^{18}F-FDG sample.
8. Describe the methods of sterilizing radioactive samples.
9. Describe the methods of sterility tests and pyrogen tests.
10. A sterile sample is always pyrogen-free. True _____; False _____.

References and Suggested Reading

1. Hamacher K, Coenen HH, Stöcklin G. Efficient stereospecific synthesis of NCA 2-[^{18}F]-fluoro-2-deoxy-D-glucose using aminopolyether supported nucleophilic substitution. *J Nucl Med.* 1986;27:235.
2. Kabalka GW, Lambrecht RM, Fowler JS, et al. Synthesis of ^{15}O-labelled butanol via organoborane chemistry. *Appl Radiat Isot.* 1985;36:853.
3. Luxen A, Guillaume M, Melega WP, et al. Production of 6-[^{18}F]fluoro-L-dopa and its metabolism in vivo—a critical review. *Nucl Med Biol.* 1992;19:149.
4. Machulla HJ, Blocher A, Kuntzch M, et al. Simplified labeling approach for synthesizing 3′-deoxy-3′-[^{18}F]fluoro-thymidine [^{18}F]FLT. *J Radioanal Nucl Chem.* 2000;243:843.
5. Mazière B, Coenen HH, Haldin C, et al. PET radioligands for dopamine receptors and re-uptake sites: chemistry and biochemistry. *Nucl Med Biol.* 1992;19:497.
6. Meyer GJ, Ostercholz A, Handeshagen H. ^{15}O-water constant infusion system for clinical routine application. *J Label Comp Radiopharm.* 1986;23:1209.
7. Saha GB. *Fundamentals of Nuclear Pharmacy.* 5th ed. New York: Springer-Verlag; 2004.
8. Stöcklin G, Pike VW, eds. *Radiopharmaceuticals for Positron Emission Tomography.* Dordrecht, The Netherlands: Kluwer Academic:1993.
9. U.S. Pharmacopeia 26 & National Formulary 21. United States Pharmaceutical Convention, Rockville, MD; 2003.
10. Welch MJ, Kilbourn MR. A remote system for the routine production of oxygen-15 radiopharmaceuticals. *J Label Comp Radiopharm.* 1985;22:1193.
11. Wieland D, Bida G, Padgett H, et al. In-target production of [^{13}N]ammonia via proton irradiation of dilute aqueous ethanol and acetic acid mixtures. *Appl Radiat Isot.* 1991;42:1095.

8
Regulations Governing PET Radiopharmaceuticals

The use of PET radiopharmaceuticals is regulated for both pharmaceutical quality as well as radiation exposure. In the USA, the pharmaceutical quality (e.g., stability, biological safety, efficacy, etc.) of PET radiopharmaceuticals is regulated by the United States Food and Drug Administration (FDA), whereas the radiation aspects are regulated by a state agency of each state. Because PET radionuclides are produced in cyclotrons and accelerators, they do not fall under the jurisdiction of the Nuclear Regulatory Commission (NRC) and are regulated by the state agency (e.g., Health Department, Environmental Protection Department, etc.). The following is a brief description of different regulations that affect the use of PET radiopharmaceuticals. Only the important points of the regulations are presented.

Food and Drug Administration

Since 1975, the clinical use of all radiopharmaceuticals has been regulated by the US FDA. For investigational purposes, a Notice of Claimed Investigational Exemption for a New Drug (IND) is submitted by a sponsor (an individual or a commercial manufacturer) to the FDA for approval of the protocol to use a specific radiopharmaceutical in humans. There are three phases in the IND clinical investigation of a radiopharmaceutical. In Phase I, only pharmacologic and biodistribution data of the radiopharmaceutical are obtained in a limited number of humans and no therapeutic and diagnostic evaluation can be made. In Phase II, clinical effectiveness of the radiopharmaceutical is evaluated for a specific disease only in a few patients. In Phase III, a large number of patients are included in the clinical trial to establish the safety and clinical effectiveness of the radiopharmaceutical for a specific disease.

After a radiopharmaceutical is proven by clinical trials to be safe and efficacious for a specific clinical indication, a New Drug Application (NDA) is submitted with all clinical data by a commercial vendor to the FDA for approval to market it. If the FDA is convinced of the safety and effectiveness of the radiopharmaceutical for a clinical indication, the FDA then approves the product for marketing. It takes a long time (at times, a couple of years) from IND to NDA for approval of a particular radiopharmaceutical for clinical use in humans.

PET radiopharmaceuticals are uniquely different from conventional radiopharmaceuticals because they are short-lived and most are produced on site at the cyclotron facility. In most cases, synthesis of these tracers by radiolabeling with positron emitters is accomplished by online automated methods for the sake of brevity. Several lengthy quality control tests are performed on an "after-the-fact" basis. The production methods and their technical details may vary from facility to facility. For these reasons, the FDA treats PET radiopharmaceuticals somewhat differently and attempts to standardize the techniques employed in all facilities. In 1995, the FDA published in the Federal Register the following documents regarding the manufacture of PET radiopharmaceuticals: (1) Regulation of Positron Emission Tomography Radiopharmaceutical Drug Products: Public Workshop: February 27, 1995, 60 Fed.Reg. 10594; (2) Draft Guideline on the Manufacture of Positron Emission Tomography Radiopharmaceutical Drug Products; Availability: February 27, 1995, 60 Fed.Reg. 10593; (3) Current Good Manufacturing Practice for Finished Pharmaceuticals; Positron Emission Tomography: April 22, 1997, 62 Fed.Reg. 19493. These regulations provided guidance for submission of NDAs and abbreviated NDAs (ANDAs) for PET radiopharmaceuticals to the FDA, and the guidelines gave details of the current good manufacturing practice (CGMP) to follow in the manufacture of PET radiopharmaceuticals.

However, the above regulations and guidelines were considered to be costly and burdensome by the nuclear medicine community, particularly the commercial vendors. Also, other radiopharmaceuticals as well as conventional drugs were subjected to strict scrutiny by the FDA, resulting in a very long waiting time for marketing approval. Following strong lobbying by the nuclear medicine community, drug manufacturers, and other stakeholders, the US Congress enacted the FDA Modernization Act (FDAMA) (Public Law 105–115) in 1997 to overhaul several aspects of the drug manufacturing industry, which took effect on November 21, 1997. Under the Act, the above three regulations regarding PET radiopharmaceuticals were retracted and new provisions were introduced.

In the FDAMA, PET radiopharmaceuticals are categorized as positron-emitting drugs compounded by, or on the order of, a licensed practitioner following the state's regulations, and meeting the specifications of the official monographs of the USP. The FDAMA directed the FDA to develop approval procedures and guidance for the manufacture of PET radiopharmaceuticals within a time frame of four years. In this four-year time line, all PET tracer-producing facilities in the United States were to be registered as drug manufacturers. In the first two years, the FDA was to consult with patient advocacy groups, professional associations, manufacturers, physicians, and scientists who prepare or use PET drugs in developing approval procedures and CGMP for PET radiopharmaceuticals. The remaining two years were allowed for all PET radiopharmaceutical manufacturing facilities to comply with the new PET drug CGMP and register as manufacturers. During these four years, the FDAMA prohibited the FDA to require the submission of NDAs or ANDAs for PET radiopharmaceuticals produced according to the USP specifications. However, voluntary submissions of NDAs or ANDAs were not prohibited.

Under the mandate of the FDAMA, the FDA issued in the Federal Register a notice entitled, "Positron Emission Tomography Drug Products: Safety and Effectiveness of Certain PET Drugs for Specific Indications" (March 10, 2000, 65 Fed.Reg. 12999). In this notice, the FDA concluded that certain PET radiopharmaceuticals, when produced under specific conditions, are safe and effective for certain clinical indications. The three PET radiopharmaceuticals considered in the notice were ^{18}F-sodium fluoride for bone imaging, ^{18}F-FDG for use in oncology and for assessment of myocardial viability, and ^{13}N-NH$_3$ for evaluation of myocardial blood flow. The evaluation of these radiopharmaceuticals was based on literature reviews by the FDA as permitted under Section 505 of the FDAMA. This is in contrast to conventional NDA approval, in which the safety and effectiveness of a drug are typically demonstrated in experiments by the applicant.

It should be noted that ^{18}F-sodium fluoride was approved by the FDA in 1972 for bone imaging, but marketing was stopped by the NDA holder in 1975. Basically, the current approval of ^{18}F-sodium fluoride is a reactivation of an already approved NDA. ^{82}Rb-rubidium chloride was approved by the FDA for evaluation of myocardial perfusion in 1989, and in 1994 the FDA approved an NDA submitted by the Methodist Medical Center of Illinois for ^{18}F-FDG injection to evaluate abnormal glucose metabolism in epileptic foci.

The FDA also published in the Federal Register a draft guidance for industry entitled, "PET Drug Applications—Content and Format for NDAs and ANDAs" (March 10, 2000, 65 Fed.Reg. 13010). It is intended to assist manufacturers of certain PET radiopharmaceuticals in submitting NDAs or ANDAs, in accordance with the notice entitled, "Positron Emission Tomography Drug Products, Safety and Effectiveness of Certain PET Drugs for Specific Indications," mentioned above. Comments were solicited until a final rule is adopted. The guidance details the criteria for when to apply for an NDA or an ANDA, and what to include in the application.

As mandated by the FDAMA, the FDA issued on April 1, 2002 in the Federal Register a preliminary draft proposed rule on current good manufacturing practice for PET radiopharmaceuticals (April 1, 2002, 67 Fed.Reg. 15344). Along with it, the FDA also published a draft guidance entitled, "PET Drug Products—Current Good Manufacturing Practice (CGMP)" (April 1, 2002, 67 Fed.Reg. 15404). The FDA solicited public comments on both these instruments and held a public meeting on May 21, 2002. However, no final rule or guidance has been issued as yet.

Whereas readers are referred to these specific documents for details available on the website www.fda.gov/cder/fdama, some of the specifics are briefly mentioned here. The essence of these two documents emphasizes the importance of the overall quality assurance in manufacturing a PET radiopharmaceutical. All equipment and measurements used in the manufacture must be validated. The areas and hoods in which PET radiopharmaceuticals are manufactured must be run in a sterile condition. The personnel responsible for the manufacture must be well trained in the methodology, and an appropriate number of personnel are required in a production laboratory. Each step of the production must be verified and records must be maintained. The sterility and pyrogen testing of the finished product must be performed by appropriate methods. If a PET radiopharmaceutical is to be commercially distributed, appropriate containers and techniques must be adopted for safe shipments.

At the time of this writing, the manufacture of PET radiopharmaceuticals is under vague regulatory premise, because most of the rules and guidances are still in the draft stage. The 4-year time line mandated by the FDAMA has passed more than three years ago, yet no definite regulations have been implemented for PET radiopharmaceuticals. It is anticipated that final rules will be established soon by the FDA to the satisfaction of the nuclear medicine community. In the meantime, the manufacturers can produce PET radiopharmaceuticals following the specifications of the official monographs of the USP, the guidelines of pharmacy compounding, and regulations of the state boards of pharmacy and medicine.

Radioactive Drug Research Committee

In order to expedite investigations of new radiopharmaceuticals, the FDA allows institutions to form the so-called *Radioactive Drug Research Committee* (RDRC), which functions like a mini-FDA. The Committee is composed of a nuclear physician, a radiochemist or radiopharmacist, an RSO, and at least two more individuals of other disciplines, and is primarily charged with the approving and monitoring of protocols involving the investigational use of radiopharmaceuticals in humans. Under this category, the study cannot be used for diagnostic and therapeutic purposes; only pharmacokinetic data (biodistribution, absorption, metabolism, and excretion) can be obtained; the radiation dose to the critical organ cannot be more than 3 rem (0.03 Sv) from a single dosage, and a total of greater than 5 rem (0.05 Sv) per year during the entire study; and only 30 patients can be studied per protocol. The RDRCs are very helpful in investigations with PET radiopharmaceuticals, obviating need for an IND with the FDA.

The RDRCs are approved by the FDA, and an annual progress report must be submitted to the FDA.

Radiation Regulations for PET Radiopharmaceuticals

Whereas the NRC regulates only the reactor-produced radionuclides, the state agencies (e.g., Health Department, Environmental Protection Department, etc.) regulate the accelerator-produced or cyclotron-produced radionuclides. At the time of this writing in the United States, 33 of the 50 states have entered into agreement with the NRC to regulate the reactor-produced radionuclides as well. They are called the Agreement states and implement all NRC regulations for reactor-produced radionuclides along with the regulations of accelerator- or cyclotron-produced radionuclides. Accordingly, the states (both Agreement states and NRC states) regulate PET radiopharmaceuticals, since PET radionuclides are produced in the cyclotron. Regulations vary among the 50 states, but the basic principles of radiation regulations are the same for all states. Given below are the highlights of some important and pertinent regulations concerning the clinical and research use of PET radiopharmaceuticals.

License or Registration

Facilities: The PET center and/or the cyclotron facility must be registered or licensed by the state for the production or use of PET radiopharmaceuticals. The license for medical use of radiopharmaceuticals is called the radioactive material (RAM) license, which a licensee obtains after applying to the state. The RAM license specifies the type, chemical form, and the possession limit of the radionuclides to be used, depending on the scope of the operation at the applicant's facility. While a PET center may be approved for a few hundred millicuries of ^{18}F-FDG in its RAM license, the cyclotron facilities may be approved in the license for curie amounts for commercial distribution. Note that the ^{82}Sr-^{82}Rb generator typically is supplied in a strength of 80 to 150 mCi (2.96 to 5.55 GBq) of ^{82}Sr, but it also contains ^{85}Sr which may be as much as five times the amount of ^{82}Sr. Although ^{85}Sr is not used clinically, but is contained in the generator, a licensee has to include in the RAM license the maximum possible amount of ^{85}Sr as the possession limit in addition to those of ^{82}Sr and ^{82}Rb. These licenses are issued for a certain number of years (e.g., 1 year, 3 years, etc.), which varies from state to state, and renewed after the period, if needed. The licensee agrees in the license application to strictly follow all the terms and regulations implemented by the state.

A cyclotron is required to be registered with the state since it produces radionuclides. A dedicated PET scanner may or may not be required to be registered in a state depending on the state's statutes on this matter. Many states require a certificate of need (CON) prior to the purchase of a PET scanner, a mobile PET, or a PET/CT scanner. A PET/CT scanner is required to be registered with the state because of the CT unit, since all states require registration of radiation-generating machines.

Physicians: All states require some form of licensing of physicians to use radioactive materials in humans. Following the requirements of the NRC (10CFR35.290), the states may require physicians to have similar training and experience to be authorized users for the cyclotron-produced radionuclides. In these cases, accredited board certifications or minimum hours of training and experience are required to qualify as authorized users. As required by the NRC, 700 hours of training and experience, which include classroom and laboratory training in radiation science and work experience in radioisotope handling, would be needed to qualify as an authorized user for imaging and localization studies using PET radiopharmaceuticals (10CFR35.290). In addition to training and work experience, a preceptor's certification as to the competence of the individual is required. The specialty boards that meet the requirements of the above hours of training and work experience are considered for authorization.

Technologists: To work in nuclear medicine in the United States, a nuclear medicine technologist is required to be certified by the Nuclear Medicine Technology Certification Board (NMTCB) or the American Registry of Radiologic Technologists (ARRT) with specialty in nuclear medicine technology. Many states require healthcare technologists to be licensed to practice their profession in the state. At present, 22 states in the country require licensing for nuclear medicine; 38 states require licensure for radiographers; and 32 states require licensure for radiation therapists. Congress is considering the passage of the Consumer Assurance of Radiologic Excellence (CARE) bill to establish educational and credentialing standards for personnel who perform medical imaging and radiation therapy procedures. The nuclear medicine technology licensure is given based on the NMTCB certification and work experience. The duration of the license varies among the states, but they are renewable on the accrual of required continuing medical education (CME) credits. Current nuclear medicine technologists can work as PET technologists; however, many consider PET technology to be a unique modality, and hence see a need for a separate certification for the PET technologists. The NMTCB introduces a PET specialty examination starting in 2004 for nuclear medicine technologists, and an augmented version of the PET specialty examination beginning in 2005 for registered radiographers and radiation therapy technologists.

The PET/CT units involve the use of two modalities—PET using radionuclides and CT using x-ray radiations—thus complicating the issue of personnel as to who will operate them for a given patient study. Ideally, technologists credentialed in both CT and nuclear medicine technology should operate PET/CT units. However, regulations vary from state to state regarding the operation of PET/CT. Some states require dual certification of the technologists in nuclear medicine and radiography, or require two technologists—one certified in nuclear medicine and the other in radiography. A few states even require credentialing in CT through a specialty examination offered by the ARRT. About 5000 technologists nationwide are registered both in radiography by the ARRT and in nuclear medicine technology by either the ARRT or the NMCTB. Even a fewer number, about 200, are ARRT- or NMTCB-certified technologists who are also credentialed in CT by the ARRT. With such a shortage of qualified technologists, requiring dual certification is impractical, and employment of two technologists is not an economically suitable option for PET/CT operation at present.

Based on these circumstances, the Society of Nuclear Medicine Technologists Section (SNMTS) and the American Society of Radiologic Technologists (ASRT) jointly issued two consensus statements that were published in *Journal of Nuclear Medicine Technology*, 2002; 30:201. The first statement says in part, "*Any registered radiographer with the credential RT (R), registered radiation therapist with the credential RT (T), or registered nuclear medicine technologist with the credential RT (N) or CNMT may operate PET/CT equipment after obtaining appropriate additional education or training and demonstrating competency...*" A task force has been appointed by the ASRT and SNMTS to outline and recommend a formal course of study for PET/CT technologists. The second consensus statement says in part, "*States that license radiographers, nuclear medicine technologists, or radiation therapists are encouraged to amend their regulations to permit any of these individuals to perform PET/CT examinations after they have received appropriate additional education or training and demonstrate competency. States that do not currently license radiographers, nuclear medicine technologists, or radiation therapists are encouraged to adopt laws that regulate education and credentialing of these individuals...*" Following these consensus statements, the ARRT will offer an augmented ARRT/CT certification for PET/CT operation to nuclear medicine technologists certified by the ARRT or NMTCB.

As it stands now, in states requiring dual certification, two technologists—one certified for the CT part and the other for the PET part—must be employed to perform the PET/CT procedure, unless the technologist is certified in both modalities. In other states, a registered nuclear medicine technologist should be able to perform both PET and CT as long as the technologist is competent in both modalities.

Regulations for Radiation Protection

Because radiation causes damage in living systems, international and national organizations have been established to set guidelines for safe handling of radiations. The International Committee on Radiological Protection (ICRP) and the National Council on Radiation Protection and Measurement (NCRP) are two such organizations. They are composed of experts in the subject of radiation, and set guidelines for working with radiation and limits of radiation exposure and dose to the radiation workers as well as the general public. The NRC or the state agencies adopt these recommendations and implement them into radiation protection programs in the United States.

Definitions

Roentgen (R) is a measure of external exposure to radiations and is defined by the amount of γ or x-ray radiation that produces 2.58×10^{-4} coulombs (C) of charge per kilogram of air. This unit applies only to air, and γ and x-ray radiations of energy less than 3 MeV.

Rad is a universal unit and is defined as

$$1 \text{ rad} = 100 \text{ ergs/gm absorber}$$
$$= 10^{-2} \text{ Joule/kg absorber}$$

In System Internationale (SI) units, it is termed *gray* (Gy) and given by

$$1 \text{ gray (Gy)} = 100 \text{ rad}$$
$$= 1 \text{ J/kg absorber}$$

Rem is the unit of dose equivalent and accounts for the differences in effectiveness of different radiations in causing biological damage. It is denoted by H and has the unit of rem. Thus,

$$H_r \text{ (rem)} = \text{rad} \times W_r$$

where W_r is the radiation weighting factor for radiation type r. W_r is related to linear energy transfer of the radiation and reflects the effectiveness of the radiation to cause biological damage.

In SI units, the dose equivalent H_r is given by *sievert* (Sv).

$$1 \text{ sievert (Sv)} = 100 \text{ rem}$$

The values of radiation weighting factors W_r for different radiations are given in Table 8.1.

Committed dose equivalent ($H_{T,50}$) is the dose equivalent to organs or tissues of reference (T) that will be received from an intake of radioactive material by an individual during the 50-year period following the intake.

Deep-dose equivalent (H_d), which applies to the external whole-body exposure, is the dose equivalent at a tissue depth of 1 cm (1000 mg/cm^2).

Shallow-dose equivalent (H_S), which applies to the external exposure of the skin or an extremity, is the dose equivalent at a tissue depth of 0.007 cm (7 mg/cm^2) averaged over an area of 1 cm^2.

TABLE 8.1. Radiation weighting factors (W_r) of different radiations.

Type of radiation	W_r
x-rays, γ rays, β particles	1.0
Neutrons and protons	10.0
α particles	20.0
Heavy ions	20.0

TABLE 8.2. Tissue weighting factors, W_T, of different tissues.

Tissue	W_T^*
Gonads	0.25
Breast	0.15
Red bone marrow	0.12
Lungs	0.12
Thyroid	0.03
Bone surfaces	0.03
Remainder	0.30
Total body	1.00

* From 10CFR20.

Effective dose equivalent (H_E) is the sum of the products of the tissue weighting factors (W_T) applicable to each of the body organs or tissues that are irradiated and the committed dose equivalent to the corresponding organ or tissue ($H_E = \Sigma W_T \times H_{T,r}$). W_T accounts for the tissue sensitivity to radiation and their values are given in Table 8.2. Note that this is due to committed dose equivalent from internal uptake of radiation. This quantity is termed simply effective dose.

Total effective dose equivalent (*TEDE*) is the sum of the deep-dose equivalent (for external exposure) and the committed effective dose equivalent (for internal exposure).

Radiation area is an area in which an individual could receive from a radiation source a dose equivalent in excess of 5mrem (0.05mSv) in 1hr at 30cm from the source.

High radiation area is an area in which an individual could receive from a radiation source a dose equivalent in excess of 100mrem (1mSv) in 1hr at 30cm from the source.

Very high radiation area is an area in which an individual could receive from radiation sources an absorbed dose in excess of 500rad (5Gy) in 1hr at 1m from the source.

Restricted area is an area of limited access that the licensee establishes for the purpose of protecting individuals against undue risks from exposure to radiation and radioactive materials.

Unrestricted area is an area in which an individual could receive from an external source a maximum dose of 2mrem (20μSv)/hr, and access to the area is neither limited nor controlled by the licensee.

Controlled area is an area outside of the restricted area but inside the site boundary, access to which is limited by the licensee for any reason.

Caution Signs and Labels

Specific signs, symbols, and labels are used to warn people of possible danger from the presence of radiations in an area. These signs use magenta, purple, and black colors on a yellow background. Some typical signs are shown in Figure 8-1.

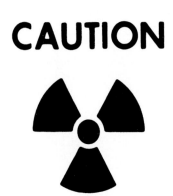

CAUTION

RADIATION

AREA

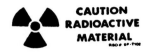

CAUTION

RADIOACTIVE MATERIAL

ISOTOPE................................

AMOUNT................................

DATE..........BY

DO NOT REMOVE THIS TAG

WITHOUT AUTHORIZATION OF

_____

CAUTION
RADIOACTIVE
MATERIAL

FIGURE 8-1. Radiation caution signs and labels.

Caution: Radiation Area: This sign must be posted in radiation areas.

Caution: High Radiation Area or Danger: High Radiation Area: This sign must be posted in high radiation areas.

Caution: Radioactive Material or Danger: Radioactive Material: This sign is posted in areas or rooms in which 10 times the quantity or more of any licensed material specified in Appendix C of 10CFR20 are used or stored. All containers with quantities of licensed materials exceeding those specified in Appendix C of 10CFR20 should be labeled with this sign. These labels must be removed or defaced prior to disposal of the container in the unrestricted areas.

Radiation Safety Officer

Large institutions employ radiation safety officers (RSOs) to implement and monitor various regulations for the use of radioactive materials. Smaller facilities such as clinics and standalone units often appoint authorized users as RSOs and hire an outside firm, which advises and monitors the radiation safety program at the facility. In these facilities, a radiation safety committee (RSC) is not needed. The duties of an RSO include investigations of accidents, spills, losses, thefts, misadministrations, unauthorized receipts, uses, and transfers of radioactive materials and instituting corrective actions. In larger institutions, in addition to the RSO, an RSC is required, which is composed of individuals experienced in radiation safety and oversees the overall radiation protection program at the institution. The

RSO works with the recommendations of the RSC in setting the policies and procedures for the purchase, receipt, storage, transfer, and disposal of the radioactive materials. The RSO conducts periodic checks of calibration of survey instruments, dose calibrators, and surveys of radiation areas, and keeps records of all activities related to the use of radiation at the facility.

Occupational Dose Limits

The annual occupational dose limit to an adult radiation worker is the more limiting of (1) total effective dose of 5 rem (0.05 Sv) or (2) the sum of deep dose equivalent and the committed dose equivalent to any individual organ or tissue, other than the lens of the eye, being equal to 50 rem (0.5 Sv).

The limit on the annual occupational dose to the lens of the eye is 15 rem (0.15 Sv).

The limit on the annual occupational dose to the skin and other extremities is the shallow dose equivalent of 50 rem (0.5 Sv).

The annual occupational effective dose limit for the minor (<18 yrs working with radiation) is 0.5 rem (5 mSv). The occupational dose limit to the embryo/fetus during the entire gestation period of a declared pregnant radiation worker is 0.5 rem (5 mSv) with a monthly limit of 0.05 rem (0.5 mSv).

The effective dose to an individual member of the public is limited to 0.1 rem (1 mSv) per year.

Personnel Monitoring

Personnel monitoring is required when an occupational worker is likely to receive in excess of 10% of the annual dose limit from radiation sources, and for individuals entering high or very high radiation areas. Monitoring is accomplished by using film badges or thermoluminiscent dosimeters (TLD).

The film badge is the most common method of personnel monitoring because of its cost effectiveness. It gives reasonably accurate readings of exposure from β, γ and x-ray radiations. The film badge consists of radiation-sensitive film held in a holder. Filters of different materials (aluminum, copper and cadmium) are attached to the holder in front of the film to differentiate the exposures from radiations of different energies and types. The density of the film changes with exposure to radiation and is measured after development by a densitometer. The measured density is proportional to the exposure from the radiation. The film badges are changed monthly and therefore give integrated radiation dose to the worker for every month.

The TLD consists of inorganic crystals of lithium fluoride (LiF) or manganese activated calcium fluoride (CaF_2:Mn) held in holders, and is commonly used for finger exposures. TLDs exposed to radiations emit light when heated at 300° to 400°C and the amount of light is proportional to radiation energy absorbed, thus giving the exposure value. The TLD readings are reasonably accurate.

Receiving and Monitoring of Radioactive Packages

All packages carrying radioactive material are required to be monitored for possible radioactive contamination. Even though PET radiopharmaceuticals do not fall under the realm of the NRC, the regulations described in 10CFR20 of the NRC are the plausible guide for monitoring the received radioactive packages and states normally follow this guide. Monitoring should be done within 3 hours of delivery if the package is delivered in normal working hours, or no later than 3 hours from the beginning of the next working day if it is received after working hours.

Two types of monitoring are performed: survey for external exposure and wipe test for removable contamination on the surface of the package due to possible leakage of the radioactive material. The external survey is conducted by using a Geiger-Müller (GM) survey meter at the surface and at 1 meter from the package. The wipe test for removable contamination is carried out by swabbing three 100cm^2 areas on the package surface using absorbent paper and counting the swabs in a NaI(Tl) well counter. The NRC limits of these measurements are:

Tests	Limits
survey at the surface	$\leq 200\text{mR/hr}$
survey at 1 meter	$\leq 10\text{mR/hr}$
wipe test	$\leq 6600\text{dpm}/300\text{cm}^2$

If any of the readings exceeds the limit, the carrier and the Radiation Safety Officer should be notified for further corrective action. All the data of monitoring are recorded in a logbook (Figure 8-2).

ALARA Program

Although regulations allow an annual maximum permissible dose to radiation workers, one should make considerable efforts to adopt strict protective measures in working with radiations so as to reduce the radiation dose *as low as reasonably achievable* (ALARA). Under this concept, techniques, equipment, and procedures are critically evaluated and adopted to minimize the radiation dose to the worker. The NRC has set two goals for a radiation worker to achieve: 10% of the occupational dose per quarter (Action level I) and 30% of the occupational dose per quarter (Action level II). If these limits are exceeded, corrective action must be taken or higher limits must be justified for a particular situation. Even though PET radiopharmaceuticals do not fall under the NRC, these values are accepted by states as a suitable guide for ALARA principles to adopt in PET facilities.

¹⁸F-FDG RECEIPT AND USE RECORD
(UNIT DOSE)

Date	Mfr.Name	Rx. No	*Survey(mR/hr) At Surface At 1 Meter	Wipe Test + or -	Tech Name	Vol.	Calib Dose	Calib. Time	Patient's Name	I.D. No.	Study	Act.** (Disp.)	Time of Injection	Name

Limits: GM reading at the surface = 200 mR/hr   * If the wipe test and/or survey reading exceeds the limit, contact the Radiation Safety Officer
GM reading at 1 meter = 10 mR/hr   ** All residual activity is disposed of according to regulations
Wipe test limit = 6600 dpm/300 cm²

FIGURE 8-2. A sample log sheet for record keeping of unit dosages of ^{18}F-FDG.

Radioactive Waste Disposal

Radioactive waste generated in PET facilities contain mostly short-lived radionuclides and is disposed of by the most common method of decay-in-storage. The solid waste is packaged in a yellow bag properly labeled with the date, radionuclide and level of activity (in mR), and stored for decay. When the activity level in the bag is equal to or less than the background, the yellow bag is repackaged into a black plastic bag, which is then discarded in the regular trash. Obviously, waste from ^{11}C, ^{13}N, and ^{15}O does not need to be stored for decay-in-storage because of the short half-lives and needs only to be discarded at the beginning of the next day at the latest. ^{18}F-FDG waste may need to be stored for decay depending on the level of activity and the time of the day when it is stored. For ^{82}Rb, whose half-life is only 75 seconds, its disposal is not a concern. However, ^{82}Sr ($t_{1/2} = 25.6$ days) and ^{85}Sr ($t_{1/2} = 65$ days) breakthrough in the ^{82}Rb eluate obtained for daily calibration of the ^{82}Sr-^{82}Rb generator for radiochemical yield must be monitored carefully and discarded according to the method recommended by the Radiation Safety Officer at the PET facility.

Surveys for Radiation Exposure and Contamination

Working areas, benches, equipment, etc. may be contaminated unknowingly and should be surveyed frequently to avoid unnecessary radiation exposure. Surveys for ambient radiation exposure must be performed in all work areas at the end of the day using a Geiger-Müller (GM) counter. For each area, a trigger level is established from the average of several survey readings taken over a period of time. Daily survey reading should not exceed the trigger level, but if it exceeds, the source of excess radiation is identified and corrective action should be taken.

Wipe tests should be carried out to identify any removable contamination. These tests are done by swabbing the area with absorbent paper and counting the swab in a NaI(Tl) counter. For PET radiopharmaceuticals, these readings should be less than 20000 dpm /100 cm^2 in the radiation areas at the PET facilities and 2000 dpm/cm^2 in the unrestricted areas. If the readings exceed the limits, the area or the spot must be decontaminated. These tests should be done once a week.

Syringe and Vial Shields

Since PET radionuclides produce high energy 511 keV annihilation radiations, vials and syringes containing them should be handled using appropriate lead shields. A variety of syringe shields and vial shields for PET radiopharmaceuticals are available from commercial vendors. A typical PET syringe shield and a syringe holder are shown in Figures 8-3 and 8-4. Both the syringe or syringe shield and the vial shield should be labeled conspicuously, indicating the name of the radiopharmaceutical, quantity of the activity and the date and time of calibration.

Use of Dose Calibrator

An accurate dose calibrator is needed to assay the dosage of a PET radiopharmaceutical for administration to humans. The dose calibrator must be calibrated for constancy, accuracy, linearity and geometry. The readers are referred to the reference of Saha (2004) for the details of calibration of the dose calibrator. The activity of a dosage contained in a syringe is measured

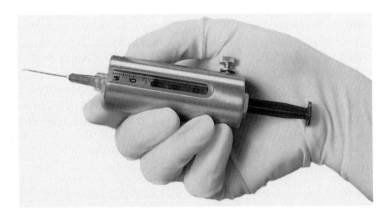

FIGURE 8-3. Lead syringe shield (Photo courtesy of Biodex Medical Systems Inc., NY.)

FIGURE 8-4. A PET syringe holder (Photo courtesy of Biodex Medical Systems Inc., NY.)

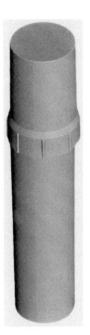

by placing the syringe in an plastic insert which is placed inside the dose calibrator. The activity is displayed in Ci, mCi, or μCi units or GBq, MBq, or kBq units. Unit dosages (e.g., ^{18}F-FDG) supplied by the manufacturers are not required to be assayed again at the receiving facility. However, it is a good idea to assay it anyway.

Radioactive Spill

It is likely in a PET facility that a radioactive spill may occur, and appropriate action must be taken. A radioactive spill may be major or minor depending on the nature and extent of contamination involved in the spill. In the case of a major spill where the spread of contamination is large or personnel are contaminated, the incident must be reported immediately to the Radiation Safety Officer. In all spills, the principle is to contain the radioactivity, and access to the area should be restricted. Cleaning the contaminated area by wiping with absorbent paper and using decontaminating liquid (Radiacwash) is all that is needed in most cases. Surveys and wipe tests must be conducted to assess the level of decontamination. In case of nonremovable contamination, a thin foil-type lead shield may be used to cover the area until the activity decays below the trigger level.

Record Keeping

Records must be maintained for the receipt, storage, dispensing, and disposal of all radioactive materials in a PET facility. All patient dosages administered to patients must be logged in a record book with the patient's name, ID number (e.g., clinic number), date and time, and quantity of the activity administered (Figure 8-2). Also, all the survey data must be recorded.

Principles of Radiation Protection

The cardinal principles of radiation protection from external radiation sources are governed by 4 factors: time, distance, shielding, and activity.

Time

The radiation dose to an individual from an external source is proportional to the time the person is exposed to the source. The longer the exposure, the higher the radiation dose. It is advisable to spend no more time than necessary near radiation sources.

Distance

The radiation exposure varies inversely with the square of the distance from the source. Each radionuclide has an exposure rate constant, Γ, which is given in units of R-cm^2/mCi-hr at 1 cm or in SI units, μGy-m^2/GBq-hr at 1 meter, and these values for ^{11}C, ^{13}N, ^{15}O, ^{18}F, and ^{82}Rb are given in Table 8.3. The exposure X per hour at distance d (cm) from an n mCi source is given by

$$X = \frac{n\Gamma}{d^2} \tag{8.1}$$

where Γ is the exposure rate constant of the radionuclide. Working at maximum possible distance from radiation is prudent in reducing radiation exposure.

Problem 8.1

Calculate the cumulative exposure a radiation worker receives from a 15 mCi (555 MBq) ^{18}F-FDG source while standing for 2 hour at a distance of 2 meters. (Γ for ^{18}F-FDG is 6.96 R-cm^2/mCi-hr at 1 cm).

TABLE 8.3. Exposure rate constants of common positron-emitting radionuclides.

Radionuclide	Γ (R-cm^2/mCi-hr at 1 cm)	Γ (μGy-m^2/GBq-hr at 1 meter)
^{11}C	7.18	193.7
^{13}N	7.18	193.7
^{15}O	7.18	193.7
^{18}F	6.96	187.9
^{82}Rb	6.10	164.9

Answer:

Since $t_{1/2}$ of ^{18}F is 1.83 hour and the worker stands for 2 hour, the activity of ^{18}F-FDG decays considerably, and hence the cumulative activity for 2 hour is calculated as follows:

$$\lambda \text{ for } {}^{18}\text{F is } 0.693/1.83 = 0.3787 \text{ hr}^{-1}$$

$$\text{The cumulative activity } A_t = A_0 \frac{1 - e^{-\lambda t}}{\lambda}$$

$$= \frac{15 \times (1 - e^{-0.3787 \times 2})}{0.3787}$$

$$= 21.04 \text{ mCi} - \text{hr}$$

Using Eq. 8.1, the cumulative exposure X at 2 meters

$$X = \frac{21.04 \times 6.96}{(200)^2}$$

$$= 0.00366 \text{ R}$$

$$= 3.66 \text{ mR}$$

Shielding

Radiations passing through absorbers lose energy by interaction with absorber material. This loss of energy is very effective in high Z materials such as lead, tungsten, etc. Therefore, these high Z materials are conveniently used as shielding materials for radiations, and lead is the shielding material of choice in most cases because it is the least expensive. Bricks, syringe shields, L-blocks (Figure 8-5), and syringe containers made of lead are common examples of shielding. Handling radioactivity behind the lead shield, using syringe shields, and carrying dosages in lead containers, etc. are typical examples of radiation protection by shielding. The concept of half-value layer (HVL) of absorbing materials for different radiations has been discussed in Chapter 1 and should be kept in mind in handling radioactivity. In PET facilities, 511 keV photons from positron emitters are highly penetrating and, therefore, larger amounts of shielding material are needed in all aspects of radiation protection.

Problem 8.2

If the HVL of lead for 511 keV photons of ^{18}F is 0.55 cm, calculate the thickness of the lead shield required to reduce the exposure by 90% from a 20 mCi ^{18}F-FDG dosage in a vial.

Answer:

According to Eq. (1.19), linear attenuation coefficient,

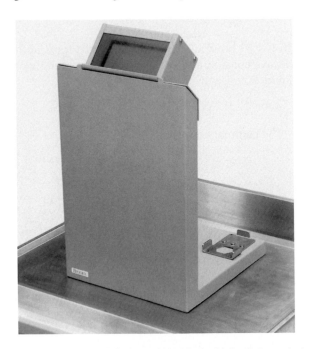

FIGURE 8-5. Lead barrier shield (L-block), behind which all formulation and han-dling of radioactive materials are carried out. (Photo courtesy of Biodex Medical Systems Inc., NY.)

$$\mu = \frac{0.693}{HVL}$$
$$= \frac{0.693}{0.55}$$
$$= 1.26 \text{ cm}^{-1}$$

Because the initial beam is reduced by 90%, the transmitted beam is 10%.

$$0.1 = 1 \times e^{-1.26xx}$$
$$\ln(0.1) = -1.26xx$$
$$2.303 = 1.26xx$$
$$x = 1.82 \text{ cm}$$

Thus, 1.82 cm of lead will be needed to reduce the exposure from a 20 mCi dosage by 90%.

Note that the 20 mCi dosage does not come into calculation because 90% reduction remains the same regardless of the quantity of dosage. However, the absolute exposure value in roentgen will depend on the dosage. The exposure X beyond the 1.82 cm lead shield is calculated using Eq. (8.1):

$$X = \frac{0.1 \times 20 \times 6.96}{(1.82)^2}$$
$$= 4.2\,R/hr$$

Activity

Understandably, the lesser amount of radioactivity will result in less radiation exposure and dose. One should use only a necessary amount of radioactivity.

Do's and Don'ts in Radiation Protection Practice

Do wear laboratory coats and gloves when working with radioactive materials.

Do work in a ventilated fumehood while working with volatile material.

Do handle radioactivity behind a lead barrier shield, such as L-block.

Do cover the trays and workbench with absorbent paper.

Do store and transport radioactive material in lead containers.

Do wear a film badge while working in the radiation laboratory.

Do identify all radionuclides and dates of assay on the containers.

Do survey work areas for contamination as frequently as possible.

Do clean up spills promptly and survey the area after cleaning.

Do not eat, drink, or smoke in the radiation laboratory.

Do not pipette any radioactive material by mouth.

Do monitor hands and feet after the day's work.

Do notify the radiation safety officer (RSO) in the case of a major spill or other emergencies related to radiation.

Department of Transportation

The Department of Transportation (DOT) regulates the transportation of radioactive materials and sets the regulations and guidelines for packaging, types of packaging material, limits of radioactivity in a package, and exposure limits for packages. All these regulations are contained in Title 49 of Code of Federal Regulations (49CFR).

The packages for radioactive shipping must pass certain tests, such as the drop test, corner drop test, compression test, and 30-minute water spray test. A special shipping container made of lead that can ship 3 unit dosages of PET radiopharmaceuticals (e.g., ^{18}F-FDG) is shown in Figure 8-6.

Radioactive packages must be properly labeled before transportation. There are 3 types of labels (Figure 8-7) based on the *transportation index*, TI, which is defined as the exposure reading in mR/hr at 1 meter from the

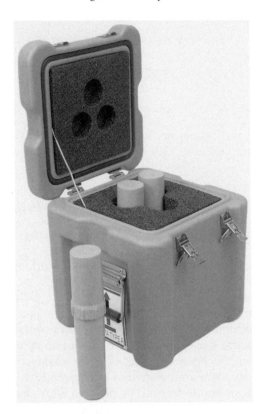

FIGURE 8-6. Special shipping containers made of lead that can ship 3 unit dosages (Photo courtesy of Biodex Medical Systems Inc., NY.)

surface of the package. The maximum permissible TI is 10. The criteria for the three labels are given in Table 8.4. The label "RADIOACTIVE" containing the value of TI must be placed on the outside of the package. For liquids, the label "THIS SIDE UP" must be pasted on the package. The label also must identify the contents and amounts of the radionuclides in

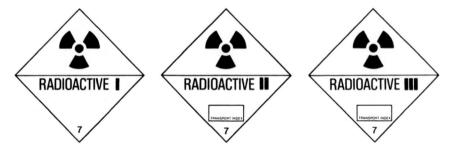

FIGURE 8-7. Three types of US Department of Transportation labels required for transportation of radioactive materials.

TABLE 8.4. Labeling categories for packages containing radioactive materials.

Type of label	Exposure (mR/hr)	
	At surface	At 1 meter
White-I	<0.5	—
Yellow-II	>0.5 ≤ 50	<1
Yellow-III	>50	>1

Note: No package shall exceed 200mR/hr at the surface of the package or 10mR/hr at 1 meter. Transport index is the reading in mR/hr at 1 meter from the package surface, and must not exceed 10.

becquerels. A shipping document containing all the above information must be placed inside the package.

According to 49CFR173.421, certain transportation requirements are exempted for radionuclides, if only a limited quantity is shipped. These limits for ^{11}C, ^{13}N and ^{18}F are 1.4mCi (or 50MBq), and those for ^{82}Sr and ^{85}Sr (for ^{82}Sr-^{82}Rb generator) are 0.54mCi (or 20MBq) and 5.4mCi (or 200MBq), respectively. The surface exposure readings should not exceed 0.5mR/hr at all points of the package surface and the wipe test measurements should be below 6600dpm/300cm^2. A notice or label, "Radioactive—Limited Quantity" must be enclosed inside or pasted outside or forwarded to the shipper along with the package. This notice must include the name of the shipper and the consignee, and the statement, "This package conforms to the conditions and limitations specified in 49CFR173.421 for radioactive material, excepted package-limited quantity of material, UN2910" in or on the package.

Employees who ship hazardous material, including radioactive material, must have hazmat training to be able to recognize and identify hazardous material, to conduct their specific functions, and to enforce safety procedures to protect the public. The training is given to a new employee within 90 days of employment and then repeated every three years. The training is provided by the employer or by other public or private sources, and a record of training must be maintained.

Distribution of ^{18}F-FDG

The need for ^{18}F-FDG is increasing tremendously as the demand for PET procedures for various clinical indications, particularly oncologic indications, increases nationwide. Although the number of cyclotron facilities is increasing in the USA, many hospitals have PET scanners but no cyclotron facility. These hospitals need ^{18}F-FDG to be supplied on a routine basis by a distant cyclotron facility.

The distribution of ^{18}F-FDG is quite challenging, because of the short half-life (110 minutes) and the distance to cover for delivery. For controlled, reliable, and economical delivery, ground shipping or air transport may be employed depending on the distance between the cyclotron facility and the PET imaging site. A maximum distance of about 200 miles may be appropriate for ground transportation, but air transport must be employed for longer distances. Air transport is risky, because of flight delay or inclement weather, and is 3 to 4 times costlier than ground transport. A dedicated charter aircraft is needed for reliable and timely delivery of ^{18}F-FDG. On the other hand, ground transportation is slower than air transport, but is more reliable. It is not as affected by inclement weather. Air transport requires delivery of ^{18}F-FDG by ground transportation from the cyclotron facility to the airport and from the airport to the client. This might negate the advantage of faster delivery by air transport.

Scheduling of delivery by ground or air transportation is the key to a successful and economically viable distribution of ^{18}F-FDG. All the orders of FDG dosages are received a day before, and deliveries to different client sites by a courier are scheduled with minimal routing. Deliveries to widely separated sites that cannot be served by one courier are made by separate couriers. Production schedule of ^{18}F-FDG batches must be synchronized with the different deliveries by separate couriers.

The shipping of ^{18}F-FDG must meet all regulations of DOT mentioned above, including approved shipping containers (DOT 7A containers, Figure 8-6) and DOT training for all FDG shippers. The interstate commercial distribution of ^{18}F-FDG requires that the vendor must obtain a license from the state to operate as a distributor.

Because of increased demand for PET procedures using ^{18}F-FDG, several commercial vendors have set up cyclotron facilities at different locations around the country and distribute ^{18}F-FDG to distant customers. PETNET, a division of CTI, has more than 3 dozen distribution centers, covering more than 50% of FDG dosages in the USA. Cardinal Health, Mallinckrodt Medical, and IBA/Eastern Isotopes have the major share of the remaining FDG sales. Many smaller suppliers as well as many academic sites are coming into the market. There were 105 FDG distribution centers in the US at the end of 2002, supplying 650 customers, compared with 400 at the end of 2001 (Burn M, 2003).

Questions

1. If a radiopharmaceutical is not approved by the FDA for clinical use, but the clinician wants to use it for investigation, what is needed from the FDA for such a situation?

2. What different aspects of PET radiopharmaceuticals are controlled by the FDA and the state or Agreement State?
3. The NRC controls the radiation aspect of PET radiopharmaceuticals. True _____; False _____.
4. The registration with the state is required for the following equipment:
   A. cyclotron   yes, no, depends on state
   B. PET/CT   yes, no, depends on state
   C. PET scanner   yes, no, depends on state
5. Review thoroughly the regulations pertaining to the practice of nuclear medicine technologists in performing PET/CT imaging.
6. Define roentgen, rad, rem, and effective dose.
7. Define restricted area, radiation area, high radiation area, and very high radiation area.
8. In a room in a nuclear medicine department, one could receive 0.15 rem (1.5 Sv) in an hour at 30 cm from the radioactive sources. What type of sign is needed on the door of the room?
9. What are the responsibilities of a radiation safety officer?
10. The occupational dose limits for radiation workers are: effective dose _____; dose to the lens of the eye _____; and dose to extremities_____.
11. The annual radiation dose limit to: (A) the declared pregnant woman during the gestation period is _____; (B) to the minor _____; and (C) to the individual member of the public _____.
12. What is the common method of personnel monitoring?
13. What are the regulatory requirements for receiving and monitoring the radioactive packages?
14. Describe the principles of ALARA program.
15. What is the most common method of radioactive waste disposal of ^{18}F-FDG in a PET facility?
16. What are the limits for the GM survey and wipe test in the laboratory where PET radiopharmaceuticals are prepared and dispensed?
17. When is personnel monitoring required of a person in a radiation laboratory?
18. Discuss the cardinal principles in radiation protection.
19. Calculate the cumulative exposure a technologist receives from a 10 mCi (370 MBq) 6-^{18}F-L-fluorodopa while standing for 2 hour at a distance of 1 meter from the source (Γ for ^{18}F is 6.96 R-cm^2/mCi-hr at 1 cm).
20. Calculate the amount of lead necessary to reduce the exposure rate from a 200 mCi ^{18}F-FDG source to less than 15 mR/hr at 30 cm from the source. (Γ for ^{18}F = 6.96 R-cm^2/mCi-hr at 1 cm; HVL of lead for ^{18}F is 0.39 cm).
21. If 1% of the primary beam exits through a patient, calculate the exposure (%) at the midline of the patient.

22. Define transport index TI. What is the maximum TI allowed by DOT for transportation of radiopharmaceuticals?
23. Elucidate the criteria for shipping "limited quantity" of radioactive material.
24. A technologist who packages and ships radioactive material must have hazmat training. True _____; False _____.
25. Does a vendor need a license from the state for interstate distribution of ^{18}F-FDG?

References and Suggested Reading

1. Burn M. PET market appears poised for continued strong growth. *Diag Imag* 2003; 25:93.
2. Federal Register, 2002; 67:15344.
3. Federal Register, 2000;65:13010.
4. Federal Register, 2000;67:12999.
5. Fusion Imaging: A new type of technologist for a new type of technology. *J Nucl Med Tech*. 2002;30:201.
6. International Commission on Radiological Protection. General Principles for the Radiation Protection of Workers. ICRP 75. New York: Elsevier; 1997.
7. National Council on Radiation Protection and Measurement. Limitation of Exposure to Ionizing, Radiation (NCRP 116). Bethesda, MD: NCRP Publications; 1993.
8. National Council on Radiation Protection and Measurements. Radiation Protection and Allied Health Personnel (NCRP 105). Bethesda, MD: NCRP Publications; 1989.
9. Nuclear Regulatory Commission. Standards for Protection Against Radiation. 10CFR part 20. Washington, DC; 1995.
10. Saha GB. *Fundamentals of Nuclear Pharmacy*. 5th ed. New York: Springer-Verlag; 2004.
11. US Food and Drug Administration. Food and Drug Administration Modernization Act of 1997. Rockville, MD, 1997.

9
Reimbursement for PET Procedures

Background

Healthcare providers (physicians, hospitals, clinics, etc.) operate and are sustained by the reimbursement or payment for care they provide. In the United States, revenue for healthcare services comes from a variety of sources including the patient, insurance companies (i.e., BlueCross/BlueShield, Cigna, Aetna), and the Centers for Medicare and Medicaid Services (CMS), formerly the Health Care Financing Administration (HCFA). The CMS provides healthcare insurance for Medicare and Medicaid beneficiaries. When interfacing with an insurance company or the CMS, there are three fundamental reimbursement concepts that must be considered to assure appropriate revenue for services provided. These include the concepts of coverage, coding, and payment.

Coverage

Coverage can be defined as the range or extent of healthcare that an insurer will pay for based on the terms of the insurance plan. Medicare has developed two pathways to secure coverage policies or guidelines for drugs and/or procedures: local coverage processes and national coverage processes. The majority of coverage decisions are made at the local level by two categories of Medicare contractors: the "fiscal intermediaries" who process claims from facilities/hospitals, and the "carriers" who process claims from physicians or freestanding imaging facilities. A National Coverage Determination (NCD) supersedes local policies and is initiated by either the request of an outside party or by the CMS. Several factors are considered when developing a national coverage determination on reimbursement for a service: 1) it meets a defined benefit category; 2) it is reasonable and necessary for the care of a patient; and 3) it is approved by the FDA for safety and effectiveness. (Some exceptions are made for products that are in clinical trials.) In addition, Medicare may request an evaluation of the health outcome of a particular procedure prior to making a national coverage decision. The CMS employs contractors, the Office of Health Technology Assessment (OHTA) in the Department of Human and Health Services, or literature reviews for the assessment of health outcome of different procedures. A national coverage decision has been developed and is currently in place for PET procedures. Private payers generally follow similar policies and procedures when establishing coverage guidelines.

Coding

CPT, HCPCS, and APC Codes

Simply defined, coding systems are used by providers and health plans to document the delivery of healthcare services for reimbursement purposes as well as to track services provided. Two major types of codes are important to consider for all clinical procedures: *Current Procedural Terminology* (CPT) codes introduced by the American Medical Association; and *Healthcare Common Procedure Coding System* (HCPCS) codes developed by a committee composed of private insurers and CMS representatives. It is important to note that the correct code to use for a service or a drug may vary based on the site of service (hospital inpatient, hospital outpatient, freestanding imaging facility) and payer type (Medicare versus non-Medicare). While HCPCS codes represent specific disease indications, CPT codes primarily describe the procedures for different clinical indications. HCPCS codes are normally used for reimbursement for PET procedures by Medicare. CPT codes can be used for indications that are not covered by Medicare.

ICD-9-CM Codes

In addition to CPT or HCPCS codes, the CMS also requires specific codes for diagnosis of diseases for inpatient, outpatient, and physician office utilization for efficient claims processing and appropriate reimbursement. These codes, called the diagnosis (Dx) codes, are listed in International Classification of Diseases, Ninth Revision, Clinical Modification (ICD-9-CM), which are based on the World Health Organization's (WHO), Ninth Revision, International Classification of Diseases (ICD-9). ICD is designed by WHO to promote international comparability in the collection, processing, classification, and presentation of mortality statistics. However, in the United States, the CMS uses similar ICD-9-CM codes for classification of surgical, diagnostic and therapeutic procedures. Along with CPT/HCPCS codes, Dx (ICD-9-CM) codes must be provided on the claim form for reimbursement. These codes are annually reviewed and updated. A new ICD-10-CM has been drafted as of July 2003, but it is not known when these revised codes will be implemented.

Payment

As with coding, payment for healthcare services also varies based on the site of service (hospital inpatient versus outpatient, physician office setting, or freestanding imaging facility) and payer type. Note that the CMS pays only for medically necessary procedures, requires precertification for specific procedures and does not pay for PET studies for screening purposes.

Hospital Inpatient Services—Medicare

Faced with the need to try to control rising hospital inpatient costs, Medicare introduced a prospective payment system known as Diagnosis Related Groups (DRG) in the early 1980s. Under the DRG program, a lump sum payment is made for all services for hospital inpatient stay based on the patient's course of hospitalization and discharge diagnosis. This payment is the same for all patients with a specific disease regardless of the length of the hospital stay.

Hospital Outpatient Services—Medicare

The CMS then focused their attention on hospital outpatient cost issues and implemented the Hospital Outpatient Prospective Payment System (HOPPS) on August 1, 2000, based on Ambulatory Payment Classification (APC) Groups. APCs are groupings of procedures that are clinically comparable and similar in terms of resource utilization. APCs are similar to the hospital inpatient DRGs in that a fixed rate is paid for a grouping of procedures based on the reported hospital costs. APCs apply to a hospital-based facility or technical fees; professional fees are paid separately. Under HOPPS, all outpatient services are grouped into APCs based on the CPT or HCPCS codes. The CMS annually evaluates reported cost figures and revises and updates the APC groupings to establish a payment schedule for the year. The payment is also adjusted for regional variations. The rate published annually by the CMS is the national rate, which must be multiplied by a locality-specific factor to take into account the geographical variations in the cost of services provided.

Currently, radiopharmaceuticals ^{18}F-FDG, ^{82}Rb-RbCl, and ^{13}N-ammonia utilized in PET procedures are eligible for separate reimbursement in addition to the technical procedure under the Medicare HOPPS.

Freestanding Imaging Center—Medicare

Since the late 1980s, Medicare has used a system identical to the physician fee schedule called the resource based relative value scale (RBRVS) to reimburse for healthcare services in freestanding facilities. Payments for different services are made by the local Medicare carriers based on relative value units (RVUs) in each of three areas: physician's work, malpractice expense and other practice overhead costs. An RVU is determined for each type of service provided and these figures are adjusted to reflect geographic cost variations. The geographically adjusted RVUs are averaged and the average is multiplied by a conversion factor (CF) to determine the total Medicare payment for a particular APC. Thus,

$$RVU \times CF = payment$$

Local Medicare carriers annually revises and updates the values of RVU and CF to establish a payment schedule for all APCs for the year. Currently, the CMS has not set the RVUs for PET studies except for G 0125 code, and local carriers set the payment rates that include the costs for radiopharmaceuticals ^{82}Rb-RbCl, ^{13}N-ammonia, or ^{18}F-FDG.

Non-Medicare Payers—All Settings

Private insurance companies have a variety of payment arrangements with providers, and prior authorization for a PET procedure may be required. Many often follow Medicare guidelines in this payment.

Billing

There are two ways of billing: component billing and global billing. In component billing, there are two components for a given PET procedure: professional and technical components, which are billed separately. The professional component is billed for the physician interpretation services, and the technical component for facility services such as equipment, personnel time, and supplies. The global billing is made for both the technical and professional services, usually applicable to freestanding outpatient imaging centers.

Claims for reimbursements must be submitted to the CMS using HCPCS or CPT codes along with Dx (ICD-9-CM) codes for all approved clinical indications. For billing purposes, G codes (HCPCS) have been assigned for PET procedures. CPT codes can be used for "denial" of reimbursement for non-covered procedures. Private payers may be billed using CPT codes, while some private payers may require the use of the CMS HCPCS codes.

Billing Process

This section describes how a billing for a given study is processed from the beginning to the end. Prior to any study performed on a patient, the demographic data of the patient including the insurance information are entered into the computer by the admitting personnel or receptionist. This becomes a part of the overall medical record of the patient and should be available in the RIS and HIS via PACS. A diagnostic or therapeutic service is performed on the patient and the corresponding CPT or HCPCS codes are entered into the computer. These codes for most studies are usually formatted into bar codes on a template. The technologist performing the examination enters its code (G codes for PET studies) into the computer by swiping the bar code on the template using a penlight. The physician then interprets the study and the report is stored. For each study, the Dx (ICD-9-CM) code is either entered by the technologist or the physician during the dictation, depending on the way it is set up at each facility.

Next, the data for each patient are forwarded electronically to the billing department, which then assembles the data into the proper format of a claim form, normally using a computer billing software. In some complicated studies, manual billing may be done and their paper records are saved. The generated bill is then sent to the insurance company or Medicare who, after proper verification of whether it meets its criteria, accepts or rejects the claim for payment. In most cases, the amount for each examination is paid by the rate set by the insurance company or Medicare, not what is billed. There are several scenarios for Medicare payment. For hospital inpatients, Medicare pays the entire amount at the DRG rate. For hospital outpatient services, Medicare sets up a payment rate for a service, which is divided into two payments—one by Medicare and the other by the patient. The ratio between Medicare and patient payments varies with different services, but tends to be 80:20. For freestanding centers, the payment rate is fixed at the ratio of 80:20, i.e., Medicare pays 80% of an eligible charge and the patient pays 20%. If the healthcare provider is in an "assignment" contract with Medicare, the patient cannot be charged more than 20% per contract agreement.

The payment by the private insurers varies depending on the contract between the insurer and the patient. These payments may be based on the usual and customary rates (UCR) set for a region, or by company-set RVU-type values, or according to the cost of the services provided. It is essential to work with the private insurers in the region to establish a reasonable payment rate for PET studies.

Rejection of a claim often arises from improper coding, incomplete billing information, and errors in demographic data of the patient entered initially. At times, insurance companies may not even notify denials, and so a follow-up by the billing personnel is required. Even if a payment is made, it may be incorrect in the amount. The resolution of nonpayment or incorrect payment may take months, if it is accomplished at all, which is quite aggravating. Electronic billing through portals such as WebMD has eliminated many of these errors and substantially improved billing and collection.

Since rejection rate for claims is around 35%, and incorrect reimbursement is about 8% to 10%, it is essential that properly trained and knowledgeable personnel staff the billing department. The reimbursement rate for PET studies is at the high end, and many PET centers are paying special attention to the billing process and employ a skilled billing individual as a special point man to concentrate on PET reimbursement.

Often the payers are not well versed in the efficacies of PET studies, and the point man should interact with them to clarify the criteria of these studies and explain to them the appropriateness of each PET study.

Healthcare financing is continually changing with time, with a decline in reimbursement, while the cost of healthcare itself is growing. It is absolutely critical to attempt to maximize collection of reimbursement for each study, and this can be achieved only through understanding of codes for each study, providing proper codes and other information in the claim form, and appropriate follow-up in the case of rejection or incorrect payment.

Chronology of PET Reimbursement

Unlike many new modalities, for which coverage decisions are made by the local carriers, all PET reimbursements are yet decided for national coverage by the CMS. Under HCPCS systems, the CMS has assigned G codes and the corresponding APC codes for all PET procedures.

While many private insurers reimbursed for PET procedures early on, it was not until mid-1990s when the CMS first considered reimbursement for PET studies. Based on the approval of ^{82}Rb-RbCl by the FDA in 1989 for myocardial perfusion studies, and after a thorough review of scientific literature, the CMS first approved reimbursement for PET scans using ^{82}Rb-RbCl for both rest and pharmacological stress studies for patients suspected of having coronary artery disease. The coverage began March 14, 1995, and is applicable to cases in which the ^{82}Rb test is used in place of, but not in addition to, SPECT, or in cases with inconclusive SPECT studies. The screening of patients for cardiac diseases was not covered by the policy.

As already mentioned in Chapter 8, in 1994 the FDA approved ^{18}F-FDG for metabolic abnormality in epileptic foci. On March 12, 2000, the FDA expanded the approval of ^{18}F-FDG as a safe and effective metabolic tracer for cardiac and several oncologic applications. Based on these FDA approvals, and after considerable review of the literature, the CMS approved reimbursement starting in January, 1998 for two oncologic indications: staging of non-small cell lung carcinoma (NSCLC) for metastasis; and characterization of solitary pulmonary nodules (SPN) for evidence of primary tumor supported by the computed tomography (CT).

In 1999, with further evidence of efficacy of ^{18}F-FDG in oncologic indications, the CMS included coverage for the PET study of three more cancers: (1) localization of recurrent colorectal tumors indicated by rising levels of carcinoembryogenic antigen (CEA) (not covered for staging); (2) staging of lymphoma confirmed by pathology and as an alternative to a gallium scan; (3) evaluation of recurrent melanoma, prior to surgery, as an alternative to a gallium scan.

Since late 2000, the CMS made a dramatic change in its approach to coverage for PET procedures, and announced a national coverage decision on PET procedures, based on a request for broad reimbursement coverage by UCLA and Duke University. This coverage request contained the summary and analysis of the literature of ^{18}F-FDG PET studies on cancer, cardiovascular disease, epilepsy, and Alzheimer's disease. In this broad coverage, reimbursement for diagnosis, staging, therapy assessment, and recurrence of lung, colorectal, melanoma, lymphoma, head and neck, and esophageal cancers was approved. Also included in this coverage was reimbursement for diagnosis for refractory seizure and myocardial viability using ^{18}F-FDG PET following inconclusive SPECT. All these new coverages were implemented in July 2001.

In the national coverage determination, the CMS agreed to make broad approval of new indications even with the accuracy and value shown only in one aspect of the disease, provided there exists sufficient evidence of these for other aspects from biology/biochemistry in clinical trials or research. This was a big step forward in the coverage approval for various PET procedures, and accordingly the CMS agreed to evaluate coverage for breast (and possibly ovarian, cervical, and uterine) cancers and Alzheimer's disease. Based on this premise, limited coverage for breast cancer was approved on October 1, 2002. Restaging of recurrent or residual thyroid cancer of follicular cell origin by ^{18}F-FDG PET and perfusion study of the heart using ^{13}N-NH$_3$ PET were covered effective October 1, 2003. On June 15, 2004, an NCD has been issued by the CMS to cover the FDG-PET studies for the diagnosis of Alzheimer's disease and fronto-temporal dementia. Note that decisions for coverage for all PET procedures thus far have been made by the CMS, and no local carrier is authorized to make decision for the coverage of these procedures.

The CMS limited the above coverage only to PET procedures that were performed using dedicated PET scanners and excluded those performed with hybrid cameras (dual-head coincidence cameras). For Medicare coverage, the dedicated PET scanners must use BGO, NaI(Tl), or other detectors of equal or superior performance characteristics and may be full-ring or partial-ring types. Under pressure by the medical community and having realized that efficacy and outcome of a procedure depends on, among other factors, the type and quality of equipment, the CMS addressed the issues of equipment used in PET procedures. Following a thorough literature survey, the CMS finally approved coverage for coincidence gamma camera-based PET procedures for some specific indications. The gamma cameras must have detectors at least 5/8 inch thick with digital electronics, and random and scatter corrections must be made for reconstruction, which must be performed by the iterative method. Note that the CMS and private insurers do not distinguish between PET and PET/CT procedures and reimbursement is identical, i.e., there is no additional reimbursement for the CT part of PET/CT procedures unless a CT study is specifically performed for the diagnosis of a particular indication without the PET examination and a claim for reimbursement is separately filed.

The current HCPCS codes used for [82]Rb-RbCl and ^{13}N-NH$_3$ PET studies for myocardial perfusion covered by the CMS are provided in Table 9.1. The current HCPCS codes and equipment used for ^{18}F-FDG PET studies for different clinical conditions covered by the CMS are listed in Table 9.2. A few current representative Dx (ICD-9-CM) codes for the diagnosis of diseases by PET studies are given in Table 9.3.

TABLE 9.1. HCPCS codes for myocardial perfusion studies using [82]Rb-RbCl and ^{13}N-NH$_3$[1,2].

Clinical condition	HCPCS code	Coverage
Heart perfusion	G0030	PET myocardial perfusion imaging (following previous PET G0030-G0047); single study, rest, or stress (exercise &/or pharmacologic)
	G0031	PET myocardial perfusion imaging (following previous PET G0030-G0047); multiple studies, rest, or stress (exercise &/or pharmacologic)
	G0032	PET myocardial perfusion imaging (following rest SPECT); single study, rest, or stress (exercise &/or pharmacologic)
	G0033	PET myocardial perfusion imaging (following rest SPECT); multiple studies, rest, or stress (exercise &/or pharmacologic)
	G0034	PET myocardial perfusion imaging (following stress SPECT); single study, rest, or stress (exercise &/or pharmacologic)
	G0035	PET myocardial perfusion imaging (following stress SPECT); multiple studies, rest, or stress (exercise &/or pharmacologic)
	G0036	PET myocardial perfusion imaging (following coronary angiography); single study, rest, or stress (exercise &/or pharmacologic)
	G0037	PET myocardial perfusion imaging (following coronary angiography); multiple studies, rest, or stress (exercise &/or pharmacologic)
	G0038	PET myocardial perfusion imaging (following stress planar myocardial perfusion) single study, rest, or stress (exercise &/or pharmacologic)
	G0039	PET myocardial perfusion imaging (following stress planar myocardial perfusion) multiple studies, rest, or stress (exercise &/or pharmacologic)
	G0040	PET myocardial perfusion imaging (following stress echocardiogram), single study, rest, or stress (exercise &/or pharmacologic)
	G0041	PET myocardial perfusion imaging (following stress echocardiogram) multiple studies, rest, or stress (exercise &/or pharmacologic)
	G0042	PET myocardial perfusion imaging (following stress nuclear ventriculogram) single study, rest, or stress (exercise &/or pharmacologic)

TABLE 9.1. *Continued*

Clinical condition	HCPCS code	Coverage
	G0043	PET myocardial perfusion imaging (following stress nuclear ventriculogram) multiple studies, rest, or stress (exercise &/or pharmacologic)
	G0044	PET myocardial perfusion imaging (following rest ECG), single study, rest, or stress (exercise &/or pharmacologic)
	G0045	PET myocardial perfusion imaging (following rest ECG), multiple studies, rest, or stress (exercise &/or pharmacologic)
	G0046	PET myocardial perfusion imaging (following stress ECG), single study, rest, or stress (exercise &/or pharmacologic)
	G0047	PET myocardial perfusion imaging (following stress ECG), multiple studies, rest, or stress (exercise &/or pharmacologic)
	Q3000[3]	Supply of radiopharmaceutical diagnostic imaging agent, ^{82}Rb-RbCl per dose. Short description: ^{82}Rb-RbCl per dose.
	A9526[3]	Supply of radiopharmaceutical diagnostic imaging agent, Ammonia N-13, per dose. Short description: Ammonia N-13, per dose

[1] From: www.cms.hhs.gov/providers/pufdownload/anhcpedl.asp
[2] APC code for all these studies is 0285.
[3] APC code for this study is 9025.

TABLE 9.2. HCPCS codes for ^{18}F-FDG PET procedures[1,2].

Clinical condition	HCPCS code	Coverage
Single pulmonary nodule	G0125	PET imaging regional or whole body; single pulmonary nodules; Short description: PET image pulmonary nodule.
	G0126	PET lung imaging of solitary pulmonary nodules, using 2-(Fluorine-18)-fluoro-2-deoxy-D-glucose (FDG), following CT or initial staging of pathologically diagnosed non-small cell lung cancer. Short description: Lung image (PET) staging.
	G0234	PET, regional or whole body for small solitary pulmonary nodule following CT or for PET initial staging of pathologically diagnosed non-small cell lung cancer; gamma cameras only. Short description: PET WhBD pulm nod; gamma cam.
Lung cancer	G0210	PET imaging whole body; full and partial-ring PET scanners only, diagnosis; lung cancer, non-small cell. Short description: PET img WhBD ring dxlung ca.
	G0211	PET imaging whole body; full and partial-ring PET scanners only, initial staging; lung cancer, non-small cell. Short description: PET img WhBD ring init lung.

TABLE 9.2. *Continued*

Clinical condition	HCPCS code	Coverage
	G0212	PET imaging whole body; full and partial-ring PET scanners only, restaging; lung cancer, non-small cell. Short description: PET img WhBD ring restag lun.
Colorectal cancer	G0163	Positron emission tomography (PET), whole body, for recurrence of colorectal metastatic cancer. Short description: PET for rec of colorectal ca.
	G0213	PET imaging whole body; full and partial-ring PET scanners only, diagnosis; colorectal cancer. Short description: PET img WhBD ring dx colorec.
	G0214	PET imaging whole body; full and partial-ring PET scanners only, initial staging; colorectal cancer. Short description: PET img WhBD ring init colore.
	G0215	PET imaging whole body; full and partial-ring PET scanners only, restaging; colorectal cancer. Short description: PET img WhBD ring restag col.
	G0231	PET imaging whole body, for recurrence of colorectal or colorectal metastatic cancer, gamma cameras only. Short description: PET WhBD colorec; gamma cam.
Melanoma	G0165	Positron emission tomography (PET), whole body, for recurrence of melanoma or melanoma metastatic cancer. Short description: PET, rec of melanoma/met ca.
	G0216	PET imaging whole body; full and partial-ring PET scanners only,diagnosis; melanoma. Short description: PET img WhBD ring dx melanom.
	G0217	PET imaging whole body; full and partial-ring PET scanners only, initial staging; melanoma. Short description: PET img WhBD ring init melan.
	G0218	PET imaging whole body; full and partial-ring PET scanners only, restaging; melanoma. Short description: PET img WhBD ring restag mel.
	G0219	PET imaging whole body; full and partial-ring PET scanners only, for non-covered indications. Short description: PET img WhBD ring noncov IND.
	G0233	PET imaging whole body, for recurrence of melanoma or melanoma metastatic cancer, gamma cameras only. Short description: PET WhBD melanoma; gamma cam.
Lymphoma	G0164	Positron emission tomography (PET), whole body, staging and characterization of lymphoma. Short description: PET for lymphoma staging.
	G0220	PET imaging whole body; full and partial-ring PET scanners only, diagnosis; lymphoma. Short description: PET img WhBD ring dx lymphom.
	G0221	PET imaging whole body; full and partial-ring PET scanners only, initial staging; lymphoma. Short description: PET img WhBD ring init lymph.
	G0222	PET imaging whole body; full and partial-ring PET scanners only, restaging; lymphoma. Short description: PET img WhBD ring resta lymp.
	G0232	PET imaging whole body, for staging and characterization of lymphoma; gamma cameras only. Short description: PET WhBD lymphoma; gamma cam.

TABLE 9.2. *Continued*

Clinical condition	HCPCS code	Coverage
Head and neck cancer	G0223	PET imaging whole body; full and partial-ring PET scanners only, diagnosis; head and neck cancer; excluding thyroid and CNS cancers. Short description: PET imag WhBD reg ring dx head.
	G0224	PET imaging whole body; full and partial-ring PET scanners only, initial staging; head and neck cancer; excluding thyroid and CNS cancers. Short description: PET img WhBD reg ring ini hea.
	G0225	PET imaging whole body; full and partial-ring PET scanners only, restaging; head and neck cancer; excluding thyroid and CNS cancers. Short description: PET img WhBD ring restag hea.
Esophageal cancer	G0226	PET imaging whole body; full and partial-ring PET scanners only, diagnosis; esophageal cancer. Short description: PET img WhBD dx esophag.
	G0227	PET imaging whole body; full and partial-ring PET scanners only, initial staging; esophageal cancer. Short description: PET img WhBD ini esopha.
	G0228	PET imaging whole body; full and partial-ring PET scanners only, restaging; esophageal cancer. Short description: PET img WhBD restg esop.
Seizure	G0229	PET imaging; metabolic brain imaging for pre-surgical evaluation of refractory seizures; full or partial-ring PET scanners only. Short description: PET img metabolic brain ring.
Heart	G0230	PET imaging; metabolic assessment for myocardial viability following inconclusive SPECT study; full or partial-ring PET scanners only. Short description: PET myocard viability ring.
	78459[3]	PET myocardial viability assessment as a primary or initial diagnosis prior to revascularization, or following an inconclusive SPECT.
Breast cancer	G0252	PET imaging, full and partial ring PET scanners only, for initial diagnosis of breast cancer and for surgical planning for breast cancer. Short description: PET imaging initial dx.
	G0253	PET imaging for breast cancer, full and partial-ring PET scanners only, staging/restaging of local regional recurrence or distant metastases, i.e., staging/restaging after or prior to course of treatment. short description: PET Image Brst Dection Recur.
	G0254	PET imaging for breast cancer, full and partial-ring PET scanners only, evaluation of response to treatment, performed during course of treatment. Short description: PET Image brst eval to tx.
Thyroid cancer	G0296	PET imaging, full and partial ring PET scanner only, for restaging of previously treated thyroid cancer of follicular cell origin following negative I-131 whole body scan. Short description: PET imge restag thyroid cancer.

TABLE 9.2. *Continued*

Clinical condition	HCPCS code	Coverage
FDG dosage	C1775[4] (generic) C9408 (brand) Medicare Hosp. outpatient FDG dosages	Supply of radiopharmaceutical diagnostic imaging agent FDG per dose 4–40 mCi.

[1] From: www.cms.hhs.gov/providers/pufdownload/anhcpcdl.asp
[2] APC code for all these studies is 1516.
[3] APC code for 78459 is 0285.
[4] For Medicare inpatient claims, or non-Medicare inpatient or outpatient claims, consider the use of the following codes to reflect a charge for the FDG dose: A4641-xx Supply of radiopharmaceutical diagnostic imaging agent not otherwise classified or 78990-xx Provision of a diagnostic radiopharmaceutical. APC code is 1775 for C1775 and 9408 for C9408.

TABLE 9.3. Examples of current diagnosis (ICD-9-CM) codes for PET studies*.

Major clinical condition	HCPCS code	ICD-9-CM code	Specific diagnosis or staging of disease
Cardiac perfusion with ^{82}Rb-RbCl	G0030– G0047	411 412 413 428	Ischemic heart disease Old myocardial infarction Angina pectoris Heart failure
Cardiac metabolism by ^{18}F-FDG PET	78459	414	Acute, chronic ischemia atherosclerosis
Cardiac metabolism by ^{18}F-FDG following inconclusive SPECT	G0230	794	Unspecified abnormal function study of cardiovascular system
Esophageal cancer	G0226– 0228	150	Malignant neoplasm of esophagus
Breast cancer (female)	G0253– 0254	174	Malignant breast cancer
Seizure	G0229	345	Epilepsy
Lung (solitary nodule)	G0125	235.7 239.1	Trachea, bronchus, and lung cancer Neoplasm of unspecified nature; respiratory system
Lung (NSCLC)	G0210– 0212	162 196.1	Trachea, bronchus, and lung cancer Intrathoracic lymph node cancer
Colorectal cancer, diagnosis	G0213– 0215	153 154	Colon cancer Cancer of rectum, rectosigmoid junction and anus
Melanomas	G0216– 0218	172	Malignant melanoma
Lymphomas	G0220– 0222	200 201 202	Lymphoma & reticulosarcoma Hodgkin's Other lymphomas
Head & neck	G0223– 0225	140–149 160 161	Lip, oral cavity, and pharynx cancer Nasal cavities, middle ear, sinus cancer Larynx cancer

TABLE 9.3. *Continued*

Major clinical condition	HCPCS code	ICD-9-CM code	Specific diagnosis or staging of disease
All above organs except heart/brain	All	235	Neoplasm of unspecified nature
All above organs except heart and brain	All	V10	Personal history of neoplasm

* The diagnosis codes are listed in broad categories, i.e., each of these codes has subcategories for specific diagnosis. These values are obtained from ftp://ftp.cdc.gov/pub/Health_Statistics/NCHS/publications/ICD-9/2003.

Disclaimer: *The codes provided in Tables 9.1, 9.2 and 9.3 are valid at the time of this writing, but are likely to change over time following rule changes by the CMS and other regulating agencies.*

Questions

1. Which federal agency is responsible for Medicare payment for health-care services?
2. Describe briefly how a Medicare payment for a particular clinical study is decided by the Centers for Medicare and Medicaid Services.
3. What are the different types of codes that need to be provided in a claim for reimbursement?
4. What is a relative value unit (RVU)?
5. Elucidate different steps taken in generating a bill for reimbursement for a study performed on a patient.
6. Name the PET radiopharmaceuticals for which reimbursements have been approved for specific clinical indications.
7. What is the minimum thickness of NaI(Tl) crystal needed in dual-head coincidence cameras for a clinical PET procedure to be eligible for reimbursement by Medicare?

References and Suggested Reading

1. Human Drugs: Positron Emission Tomography Drug Products: Safety and Effectiveness. Food and Drug Administration Notices. *Federal Register*, March 10, 2000;65:12999.
2. Keppler JS. Federal regulations and reimbursement for PET. *J Nucl Med Technol.* 2001;29:173.
3. Medicare: Hospital Outpatient Services: Prospective Payment System. Centers for Medicare and Medicaid Services Proposed Rules. *Federal Register*, August 24, 2001; 66:44671.
4. Medicare Hospital Outpatient Services: Prospective Payment System. Health Care Financial Rules. *Federal Register*, April 7, 2002;65:18433.
5. *Positron Emission Tomography (PET) Scan Medicare Coverage Issues* Manual, Section 50–36, Transmittal 136, 2001. www.cms.gov/pubforms/transmit/r136cim.pdf.

10
Design and Cost of PET Center

With increasing reimbursement for PET studies and better diagnostic utilization of the PET modality, PET centers are growing in large numbers around the country. A PET center is a designated area to accommodate one or more PET scanners and/or PET/CT scanners, a cyclotron, a radiochemistry laboratory, and administrative areas. PET centers can be either freestanding or part of a healthcare facility. Several institutions in the country have more than one PET scanner and a cyclotron. Only a few academic institutions and some commercial facilities have more than one cyclotron. Many community hospitals may have only one PET scanner in the department of radiology or cardiology and no cyclotron, and are not likely to be considered as PET centers. The description below of the design and cost estimate of a PET center is based on the clinical operation of only one PET scanner along with a cyclotron.

The design of a PET center hinges on a number of factors: site, floor loading, size of the rooms available, traffic pattern inside the building, heating and cooling, electrical and water supply, and importantly, shielding in the facility to comply with the NRC or state regulations. These factors vary from facility to facility and from equipment to equipment from various vendors. The discussion here pertains to a generic PET center with minimal requirements for these entities, and a schematic layout of a PET center is illustrated in Figure 10-1. A cost estimate for setting up and running a PET center is given later in the chapter.

Site Planning

To build a modern PET center, it is essential to have a good site planning for a smooth and efficient installation of different units, such as the scanner and the cyclotron. An architectural blueprint must be drawn before construction begins. It is difficult and costly to make revisions after the completion of the project. Since a PET center involves the use of radiation, it must comply with all regulations of the NRC or the state regarding the

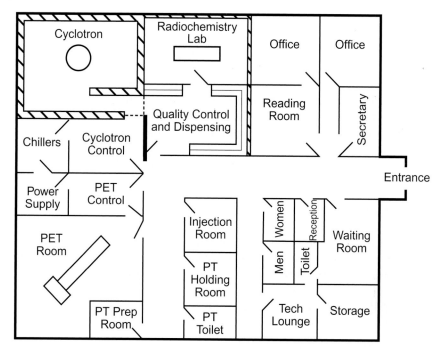

FIGURE 10-1. A schematic layout of a PET center with a cyclotron. Note that the cyclotron and PET scanner rooms are on one side and the office area is on the opposite side of the center.

exposure to the worker and the public. Logically, it is preferred to have the center far away from heavy traffic areas in the building to minimize exposure to the non-radiation worker.

It is more challenging to set up a PET center in an existing facility (such as in a nuclear medicine department) than in a totally new secluded area. Redesigning the rooms, tearing down the walls, re-routing the electrical supply, water pipes, etc. are common difficulties that are faced in modifying the existing facility to set up a PET center. Often, certain requirements may be compromised to go along with the available features at the facility. On the other hand, it is preferred and much easier to build a PET center from scratch without any compromise in requirements.

Due to the heavy weight of the shielding and magnet, the cyclotron needs to be installed on the ground floor or in the basement, and soil and underground condition must be assessed. If the water level is too shallow, or the sewer is running under, these areas should be avoided or must be supported by additional support materials. Because of relatively lighter weight, the PET scanner, however, can be installed on any strong reinforced cement floor. In seismic areas, various units need to be properly anchored in compliance with local applicable seismic codes.

Passage

Passage is an important factor to receive and bring the PET and cyclotron units inside the PET center. The hallway must be wide enough and unhindered for easy delivery of these units to the installation site. Similarly, the door to the PET or cyclotron room also should be wide enough for easy access of the delivery crates. Normally a passage of 8 × 8 feet in width and height should be optimal for the purpose. At times, in existing facilities where the current passage cannot be used, a new passage may have to be opened to allow for the delivery, thus adding to the cost.

PET Center

The PET center should be divided into three adjacent sections: one for the PET scanner facility; one for the cyclotron facilitiy; and the third for the office area. The size of the first two sections depends on the dimensions of each vendor's equipment, and the third section depends on the size and scope of the operation in a given facility.

PET Scanner Section

The PET scanner section should have six rooms: a scan room, a control room, an electronics room, a patient preparation room, an injection room, and a patient holding area. The scanner room size depends on the dimension of the PET scanner, but the variations in dimensions of scanners from different vendors are not significant. A room of 20 × 20 feet can be optimally used to install a PET scanner from any vendor, along with storage for all supplies. Under demanding circumstances, the scanner can be accommodated in smaller rooms.

Adjacent to the scan room are the electronics room for all electrical units, connecting wires, etc., and the control room where the console for the operation of the scanner is installed. There should be a glass viewing window between the scanning room and the control room for the operator to observe the patient during the study. The dimension of the electronics room should be approximately 10 feet × 8 feet and that of the control room should be about 10 feet × 10 feet. However, these dimensions can vary, if needed. All these rooms are interconnected for easy access to each room. Because the electronics modules and PET scanners generate heat during operation, cooling is essential for the equipment and a good cooling and ventilation system must be installed. There should be water supply and a sink in the PET room.

The patient preparation room should be preferably next to the above three rooms, but may be in an area not too distant from the scanner. Such a room should have a dimension of 6ft × 6ft. This room is primarily used for the patient to change for preparation for the study. This room may also be used as the injection room for administration of PET radiopharmaceuticals such as ^{18}F-FDG, if a separate injection room is not affordable.

An injection room of 6 × 6 feet should be equipped with a comfortable chair with armrest for the patient to sit on. All appropriate supplies should be stored in the room. A lead-shielded sharps container for syringe disposal and lead-shielded storage bin for other waste disposal are kept in the room.

Patients injected with ^{18}F-FDG are required to wait for 40 to 45 minutes before PET scanning and need to stay in a separate area not to cause radiation exposure to the worker or the public. The PET room, the preparation room (if it is used as an injection room), and the holding area should be well shielded to comply with the limits on radiation exposure to workers and the public. This will be discussed later in the chapter.

Cyclotron Section

The cyclotron facility should be situated at the farthest location from the inside traffic in the PET center, since its operation is not directly related to the patient and the level of radiation exposure is relatively high in this area. It should consist of minimum four rooms: cyclotron room, control room, cooling room, and radiochemistry laboratory. The size of these rooms depends on the size of equipment and space available at the facility, and they should be adjacent to each other.

The size and structural features of a cyclotron vary from vendor to vendor and so require rooms of various dimensions. A room of 25 × 25 feet should be adequate for most compact medical cyclotrons and should be equipped with a sink and floor drain. The power supply unit may be installed in the cyclotron room or in a separate room.

The weight of the magnet of a medial cyclotron runs around 22000lbs. Some cyclotrons are self-shielded with lead blocks weighing more than 35000lbs. Such heavy weight needs special consideration of the condition of the soil and the floor on which the cyclotron is to be installed. Entrance to the cyclotron room should be monitored by an electronic alarm to prevent accidental entrance to the room during the operation of the cyclotron.

The control room houses a workstation, a printer and other auxiliary terminals to operate the cyclotron. A room with the size of 10 × 10 feet should be adequate and should have easy access to the cyclotron room, but entrance must be monitored by an alarm.

The cooling system is required because of the heat generated by the electromagnet of the cyclotron and power supply unit associated with it. It consists of chillers with heat exchanger/deionizer water system that recirculates cooled water between the cyclotron and the power supply. The temperature of the system is maintained at around 7° to 15°C, depending on the type of cyclotron from a vendor. Chillers are installed in a room adjacent to the cyclotron and power supply rooms, although they are sometimes installed on the roof of the cyclotron building. The room size for chillers should be of the size 10 × 10 feet. and a floor drain is required in the room.

The radiochemistry room should be adjacent to the cyclotron for convenience of transfer of irradiated targets for processing and subsequent synthesis of PET radiopharmaceuticals. This room should be equipped with conventional labware along with a hood (preferably sterile), a sink, and steel workbench all around. The optimal size of the room should be 20 × 20 feet, and a floor drain must be installed in the room. Shielding of this room is essential because a high level of radioactivity is handled inside. To this end, the walls of this room should be thick concrete (on the order of 40 cm). The room should be well ventilated at a negative pressure and maintained at a comfortable temperature using appropriate heating and air conditioning. A section or a separate room within the radiochemistry room is designated for quality control and dispensing of PET radiopharmaceuticals.

Office Area

The office area in a PET center should have various administrative offices, a patient waiting room, a reading room, a storage room for supplies, a toilet, a file storage room, etc. The administrative offices include physicians' offices, receptionist's office, and secretary's office. Depending on the scope of the operation, the office area varies in size. In a smaller operation, all activities mentioned above are carried out in one or two rooms, while in a larger operation, many rooms are utilized for various activities for efficient operation of the PET center, as shown in Figure 10-1. The receptionist area should be in the front area of the center to receive the patients on arrival at the center. The entire area should be designed with the idea in mind that the area is an unrestricted area and so there is minimal radiation exposure not to exceed the regulatory limits from the adjacent PET scanner and the cyclotron rooms. An area between 400 and 600 square feet is an optimal estimate for the office suite in a relatively large PET center.

Caveat

A great deal of detail is involved in the planning and construction of a PET center. To insure a successful project, it is essential to have one person charged with the responsibility of managing the entire project. This person should have a strong background and experience in medical facility construction, and should be involved from the beginning to the end of the project. If such a person is not available locally, an outside planner or construction manager is recommended. This person should be the contact and liaison between the vendor and the PET center management.

As with any construction project, a construction permit must be obtained from the local authority. All local construction codes must be adhered to regarding the electricity and water supply and fire safety. A health physicist or a medical physicist should be consulted to address the issues of shielding and personnel traffic in restricted areas. A radioactive material license from the appropriate authority must be in possession for the use of PET radiopharmaceuticals, before the PET center goes into operation. Authorized physicians must be included on the license.

Shielding

A major concern in the setting up of a PET center is the shielding requirement for the walls, floors, and ceilings of the PET room, the holding room for injected patients, the cyclotron room, and the radiopharmacy room, because of the high energy 511 keV photons from positron emitters handled in these areas. As mentioned, the cyclotron should be in an area away from the inside traffic and typically is installed on the lowest floor because of the heavy weight. Also, most compact cyclotrons are self-shielded with lead blocks. Even then, the cyclotron is housed in a room with thick concrete walls to reduce the radiation exposure outside the room. An unshielded cyclotron requires a very thick concrete vault with a lengthy maze for neutron exposure reduction. The radiochemistry room is also made of thick concrete walls and normally situated away from the inside traffic. Moreover, several enclosures made of lead bricks thick enough to considerably reduce radiation exposure are utilized in the laboratory for handling the radioactivity in the synthesis of PET radiopharmaceuticals.

The shielding requirement for the PET room is somewhat different because most PET centers have a PET scanner, which is located in an area surrounded by areas often frequented by non-occupational individuals. To meet the regulatory exposure limit for these individuals, sufficient shielding in the walls and the ceiling should be provided in the PET scanner room, the injection room, and the patient holding area. It is often required to calculate how much shielding is needed to build a new PET room, or how much shielding should be added to the wall in an existing room that is to be converted to a PET scanner room. The occupational workers work mostly inside the PET suite and satisfy their radiation exposure limit of 5 rem (0.05 Sv) per year by adopting ALARA principles and all radiation protection principles within the working area. A major consideration for shielding arises for the walls, ceiling, and floor that separate the PET scanner and patient holding rooms from unrestricted areas. The radiation exposure limit for non-occupational individuals is 100 mrem (1 mSv) per year. Appropriate shielding should be estimated and provided for these areas to meet the regulatory limit. Several factors must be taken into consideration in estimating these shielding requirements, and these are discussed below.

(A) Source of radiation. The source of radiation exposure is primarily the patient injected with a PET radiopharmaceutical. The patient may be on the PET scanning table or in the holding area after injection. The PET radiopharmaceutical dosages are contained in lead-shielded containers and are not likely to contribute to the exposure.

(B) Amount of activity. The amount of activity administered to the patient determines the radiation exposure. Since the administered activity varies from patient to patient, an average value may be assumed in the estimation of shielding.

(C) Decay of activity. The activity in a patient decays over time and so radiation exposure also decreases with time from a given patient. So, how long a patient stays in the PET center determines the exposure. The exposure can be calculated from the cumulative activity integrated over time the patient stays in the holding area and the PET scanner room. Thus, the cumulative activity A_c is given by

$$A_c = A_0 \frac{1 - e^{-\lambda t}}{\lambda} \tag{10.1}$$

where A_o is the initial administered activity, λ is the decay constant of the radionuclide in question and t is the time the patient with activity stays at the facility. This time includes the time from injection to the end of scanning, i.e., the waiting time after injection (e.g., ^{18}F-FDG injection) plus the scanning time.

(D) Number of patients per day. Radiation exposure occurs when a patient is injected with radioactivity and scanned, i.e, for the duration the patient stays at the facility after injection of radiopharamaceutical. There is no exposure in the absence of a patient injected with radiopharmaceutical. Therefore, the number of patients studied per day is an important factor in calculating the shielding.

(E) Distance. The radiation exposure decreases inversely with the square of the distance between the source and the walls, floor or ceiling. The exposure X at a distance d from a point source of n mCi (MBq) activity is given by

$$X = \frac{n\Gamma}{d^2} \tag{10.2}$$

where Γ is the exposure rate constant of the radionuclide which is discussed at length in Chapter 8. The larger room cuts down the radiation exposure due to longer separation between the source and the outside of the wall.

(F) Shielding. Radiations are attenuated by absorbing material, and the attenuation depends on the atomic number and density of the material. Heavier metals such as lead, tungsten, etc. are effective shielding material to reduce radiation exposure. Construction materials such as plaster,

TABLE 10.1. Properties of different shielding materials.

Material	Atomic No (Z)	Density, ρ (g/cc)	Attenuation coeff, μ (cm^{-1})^{1,2}
Concrete	—	2.2	0.080
Iron	26	7.9	0.433
Tungsten	74	19.3	2.165
Lead	82	11.4	1.260

[1] Adapted from Towson JEC. Radiation dosimetry and protection in PET. In: Valk PE, Bailey DL, Townsend DW, Maisey MN, eds. *Positron Emission Tomography*. New York: Springer-Verlag; 2003.
[2] Based on broad beam geometry.

gypsum boards, steel and concrete have lower attenuation coefficients and thus have lesser shielding effect. The linear attenuation coefficients (μ) of some of the shielding materials are given in Table 10.1. Using these μ values, one can calculate the thickness of shielding required for an initial exposure I_o, to reduce to I_x by the following formula:

$$I_x = I_0 e^{-\mu x} \tag{10.3}$$

where I_x is the exposure beyond a thickness x of the shielding material with linear attenuation coefficient μ.

Equation (10.3) is valid for a narrow-beam geometry from a point source, and scattered radiations in the absorbing material are excluded. That is, each photon is either completely absorbed or transmitted. In reality, Compton scattering of 511 keV photons occurs within the shielding material, and some of the photons which were heading away from the location point of exposure may be scattered back toward it, thus adding to the exposure. This broad-beam geometry gives rise to what is called a *build-up factor*, B, which is given by:

$$B = \frac{\textit{Intensity of primary plus scattered radiations}}{\textit{Intensity of primary radiations only}}$$

The value of B is always greater than 1 and depends on the thickness of the shielding material. It initially increases with the thickness of the shielding material and then reaches a plateau after a certain thickness. Also, the value of B is higher in low atomic number material than in high atomic number material, due to relatively more Compton scattering in the former. Thus, the build-up factor in gypsum board is higher than in lead.

Another point of concern in using the above equation is the shape and size of the radiation source. The equation is based on the assumption of a point source of radiation, whereas in reality a patient is an extended source

TABLE 10.2. Suggested occupancy factors T^*.

Occupancy level	Type of area	T
Full	work areas, laboratories, nursing stations, living quarters, offices, children's play area	1
Partial	Corridors, restrooms, unattended parking lots	1/4
Occasional	Waiting rooms, toilets, stairways, elevators, closets	1/16

* Values suggested in NCRP 49.

of radiation. In this case, the human body can be modeled to be segmented into different sections and iterative methods can be applied to estimate the shielding requirement. Presently, a phantom called BOMAB (bottle manikin absorption) is available, simulating various regions of human anatomy (arms, thigh, abdomen, chest, head) and can be used to estimate shielding need (ANSI, 1999).

(G) Occupancy factor. The occupancy of an area refers to the amount (fraction) of time the area is occupied by an individual per week. The suggested occupancy factors T are given in Table 10.2.

Combining all the above factors, one can formulate an equation for radiation exposure as follows:

$$X = \frac{A_0 \Gamma N (1 - e^{-\lambda t}) e^{-\mu x} T}{d^2 \lambda} \tag{10.4}$$

where

X = exposure (rem or Sv per week) at distance d from the patient and beyond the thickness x of shielding material
A_o = activity in mCi (MBq) administered per patient
Γ = exposure rate constant (R-cm^2/mCi-hr at 1 cm or μGy-m^2/GBq-hr at 1 m)
N = number of patients per week
λ = decay constant (hr^{-1}) of the radionuclide
t = time (hr) the patient spends in the PET facility after receiving tracer injection
μ = linear attenuation coefficient (cm^{-1}) of photons in shielding material
T = occupancy factor for the area in question
x = thickness (cm) of shielding material

We will now illustrate an example of estimation of shielding requirements for a specific case in the design of a PET center.

Case Study

A drywall separates the PET room and a common waiting room and stands at 2 meters away from the center of the PET scanner. The facility performs six ^{18}F-FDG PET studies per day using 10 mCi (370 MBq) dosage per patient. How much shielding of lead will be needed on the wall to meet the regulatory radiation exposure limit? ($t_{1/2}$ of ^{18}F = 1.833 hr; Γ for ^{18}F = 6.96 R-cm^2/mCi-hr at 1 cm; μ for ^{18}F in lead = 1.26 cm^{-1})

The common waiting area is considered a public area, and the exposure limit is 100 mrem/year or 100 mrem/50 weeks = 2 mrem/wk.

Number of patients/wk	= 6 × 5 days/wk = 30
Activity/patient	= 10 mCi
Distance	= 2 meters or 200 cm
Patient stayed after injection	= 40 min (wait) + 20 min (scan)
	= 60 min = 1 hr
Occupancy factor for waiting room	= 1/16
Radiation exposure limit/wk	= 2 mrem/wk
	= 0.002 rem/wk
Exposure rate constant of ^{18}F	= 6.96 R-cm^2/mCi-hr at 1 cm
	= 6.96 rem-cm^2/mCi-hr at 1 cm
μ for ^{18}F in lead	= 1.26 cm^{-1}
Decay constant λ for ^{18}F	= $\dfrac{0.693}{1.833}$ = 0.378 hr^{-1}
x (thickness of shielding)	= ?

Thus,

$$0.002\,(\text{rem}/\text{wk}) = \frac{10 \times 6.96 \times 30 \times (1 - e^{-0.378 \times 1}) \times e^{-1.26 \times X}}{200^2 \times 0.378 \times 16}$$

$$= \frac{2088 \times 0.3147 \times e^{-1.26 \times X}}{241920}$$

$$e^{-1.26 \times X} = 0.7363$$

Taking logarithm,

$$-1.26 \times x = -0.306$$
$$x = 0.243 \text{ cm}$$
$$\approx 0.1 \text{ inch}$$

Thus, assuming the drywall provides no shielding, approximately 0.1 inch of lead shielding would be needed to add to the wall in order to reduce radiation exposure in the waiting area below the regulatory limit of 100 mrem/year to the public.

Cost of PET Operation

The number of PET centers is growing tremendously around the country and worldwide due to the high diagnostic value of PET in clinical medicine. In 2002, the US and worldwide sales of scanners were 334 units and 417 units respectively, compared to 267 units and 342 units in 2001 (Burn M, 2003). Because of the advantage of more accurate diagnostic value, the sale of PET/CT has outpaced that of PET alone, exceeding perhaps 80% of all sales (Waldowski, 2004) and is increasing. However, installation of PET or PET/CT units may become a financial challenge for many smaller facilities, because the recurring maintenance and support cost of PET is quite high. It is critical that a cost analysis is made to assess the financial viability of a PET operation. An article by Keppler and Conti (2001) presents an excellent cost analysis of setting up a PET center with different operational scenarios of PET scanners and a cyclotron. It is beyond the scope of this book to include such details, and only a brief estimate of the cost involved in the installation and operation of a simple PET facility is given below.

The price of a dedicated PET scanner ranges between $1 million and $1.5 million, and that of a PET/CT between $1.7 million and $2.5 million, depending on the choice of various features. The cost of construction of a PET room, a hot lab, and other ancillary spaces will be about $250,000. If the unit is to be installed in an existing facility, the cost of renovation may be even less. The hot lab and radiation safety equipment may cost another $20,000. Combining the above costs for a $1.5 million PET scanner, the total capital cost may run to $1,770,000.

A major consideration in running a PET scanner is the recurring operational cost and the volume of PET studies that can be performed. The annual cost estimate of technical operation of one PET scanner performing, say, an average of 4 patients per day is listed in Table 10.3. The total capital cost is depreciated over 5 years, giving an annual depreciation cost of $354,000. The salaries of a technologist, a receptionist, and a billing spe-

TABLE 10.3. Estimate of annual operational cost of a PET scanner (excluding professional fee)*.

Depreciation of capital cost over 5 years	$354,000
One technologist	$70,000
One receptionist	$30,000
One billing specialist	$35,000
^{18}F-FDG dosages**	$400,000
Maintenance contract (10% of the price)	$150,000
Physics service	$3,000
Casualty insurance	$6,500
Supplies and miscellaneous	$20,000
TOTAL	$1,068,500

* Based on 4 patients/day.
** Based on $400 unit dosage price of ^{18}F-FDG.

cialist are only estimates and can vary significantly in various geographical regions around the country. Assuming 4 patients/day and $400 per unit dosage of ^{18}F-FDG, the total annual cost of ^{18}F-FDG would be $400 × 4 × 250 = $400,000. The maintenance contract normally charges 10% of the price of the scanner. Many large centers having several pieces of imaging equipment often get the service contracts based on "time and material" that may lower the cost. The casualty insurance of $6,500 applies to loss of equipment by fire, flood, or other natural calamities, and the cost can vary. For freestanding facilities, a physics service from a medical physics group is needed to implement radiation safety regulations (state and/or NRC), and to keep the license current. This may cost around $3,000 per year. The total annual cost of operation adds up to $1,068,500 and the cost per patient comes out to be about $1,068. However, if the start-up money is financed, then the cost of interest per year for financing must be added. Physicians' professional compensation and cost of utilities have not been included in the analysis.

Note that the cost of $1,068 may vary from region to region in the country and at the same time, Medicare payment also is adjusted for geographical variations. The private insurers reimburse reasonably for PET procedures. Imaging facilities may have provisions for contractual write-offs and discounts. If an institution has a Medicare "assignment" agreement, the payment is limited by Medicare. Many PET centers often have a signed commitment, called the Advanced Beneficiary Notice (ABN), from the patient guaranteeing payment for the PET procedure, if the insurer declines payment. All these factors ought to be taken into consideration in the pro forma plan of a PET facility.

If a cyclotron also is planned for the PET center, then additional installation as well as recurring maintenance cost of the cyclotron must be included in the total cost estimate. At present, a medical cyclotron for 10 to 18 MeV protons would cost around $1 million to $1.2 million. Cost of the cyclotron installation and equipment for radiochemistry laboratory would run around $250,000. Depending on the scope and research programs of the PET center, a cyclotron operator, a radiochemist and a half radiopharmacist would be required for optimal operation. The combined salaries of these three individuals may cost annually $200,000 to $215,000. However, in many clinical facilities, one radiochemist assumes the responsibility of operating the cyclotron as well as synthesis of PET radiopharmaceuticals. A half radiopharmacist is needed for validation and dispensing of dosages. In parallel to the PET scanner, maintenance contract (10% of the purchase price, or "time and material" basis), casualty insurance, licensing, and supplies would add to the total operational cost. An additional item of cost is the target material for a particular PET radionuclide, which may be quite expensive depending on the enrichment and availability.

Thus, before venturing into PET business, one needs to do a thorough analysis of financial risks in the operation. What the reimbursement rate is, how well the referring physicians, particularly the oncologists, are appreciative of the effectiveness of PET procedures, whether the purchase of the PET scanner can be tied with the purchase of other equipment or service for a discount, etc. are some of the issues that need careful attention for a viable PET operation.

Questions

1. What are the different factors one should consider in designing a PET center without any cyclotron?
2. In designing a cyclotron facility, the major concern is shielding. Elaborate on different factors that must be taken into consideration in the estimation of shielding around the facility.
3. In a PET center, a clinical laboratory is situated on the other side of a plaster wall of the PET room. Calculate the amount of lead shielding required to be added to meet the regulatory limit, given the following information: number of FDG studies per week = 25; ^{18}F-FDG dosage per patient = 10 mCi; linear attenuation coefficient of 511 keV photons in lead = 1.26 cm^{-1}; Γ for ^{18}F = 6.96 R-cm^2/mCi-hr at 1 cm; distance between the scanner and the wall is 250 cm; patient stays in the department for a total of 1 hour after injection.
4. Give a cost estimate of setting up a PET center with a cyclotron in your area.

References and Suggested Reading

1. American National Standards Institute/Health Physics Society. Specifications for the Bottle Manikin Absorption Phantom (1999). McLean, VA: ANSI; ANSI/HPS N13.35; 1999.
2. Burn M. PET market appears poised for continued strong growth. *Diag Imaging.* 2003;25:93.
3. Courtney JC, Mendez P, Hidalgo-Salvatierra O, Bujenovic S. Photon shielding for a positron emission tomography suite. *Health Phys.* 2001;81:S24.
4. Kearfott KJ, Carey JE, Clemenshaw MN, Faulkner DB. Radiation protection design for a clinical positron emission tomography imaging suite. *Health Phys.* 1992;63:581.
5. Keppler JS, Conti P. A cost analysis of positron emission tomography. *Am J Roentgenol.* 2001;177:31.
6. Mathe B. Shielding design for a PET imaging suite: A case study. *Health Phys.* 2003;84:S83.
7. Waldowski K. PET/CT round table. *Advance for Imaging and Oncology.* 2004;14:28.

11
Procedures for PET Studies

In this chapter, different protocols for common PET procedures are described to provide a general understanding of how a PET study is performed. Only four procedures are included, namely whole-body imaging with ^{18}F-FDG, PET/CT whole-body imaging with ^{18}F-FDG, myocardial perfusion imaging with ^{82}Rb-RbCl, and myocardial metabolic imaging with ^{18}F-FDG. The procedures described here are generic in that there are variations in the detail of each procedure from institution to institution. Different institutions employ different techniques in immobilizing the patient on the table. Use of CT contrast agents in PET/CT is still a debatable issue, and some investigators use them, while others do not. While glucose loading is essential for myocardial ^{18}F-FDG studies in patients with low fasting glucose levels, there are varied opinions as to the lowest limit of glucose level at which glucose loading should be provided and what amount of glucose should be given orally. In lymphoma and colorectal studies, it is desirable to have a Foley catheter secured to the patient to eliminate extraneous activity in the bladder, but perhaps it is not universally employed by all.

In view of the above discussion, it is understandable that the procedures described below are a few among many with variations in detail, but the basics of PET imaging remain the same.

Whole-Body PET Imaging with ^{18}F-FDG

Physician's Directive

1. A nuclear medicine physician fills out a scheduled patient's history form indicating where the scan begins and ends on the body.
2. If the patient weighs over 250lbs, the physician authorizes a dosage of ^{18}F-FDG higher than the normal dosage.

Patient Preparation

3. The patient is instructed to fast 6 hours prior to scan.
4. Insert an IV catheter into the patient's arm for administration of ^{18}F-FDG.
5. For melanoma patients, injection must not be administered to the affected extremity. Injection should be made away from the affected area.
6. A Foley catheter is required for patients with colorectal carcinoma and lymphoma, for voiding urine.
7. Remove all metallic items such as belts, dentures, jewelry, bracelets, hearing aids, bra, etc. from the patient.
8. The patient wears a snapless gown.

Dosage Administration

9. Inject ^{18}F-FDG (10 to 15 mCi or 370 to 555 MBq in a shielded syringe) into the patient through the IV catheter.
10. The patient waits for 40 to 60 minutes with instructions to remain calm and quietly seated during this waiting period.

Scan

11. Enter patient's name, birthdate, weight, and ID number into the computer.
12. Obtain a blank transmission scan without the patient in the scanner for attenuation correction using the rotating ^{68}Ge source before the first patient is done. This blank scan is used for subsequent patients for the day.
13. After the waiting period, the patient lies supine on the scan table with the head toward the PET scanner, and with arms up or down depending on the area to be scanned.
14. Position the patient inside the scanner to the upper limit of the scan as designated by the physician. This position is marked by the computer control on the console.
15. The patient is then moved to the lower limit of the scan and the position is marked by the computer control on the console.
16. The computer determines the length of the scan field from the positions marked in Steps 14 and 15. From the manufacturer's whole-body scanner chart, determine the number of bed positions needed for the length of the scan field.
17. Enter into the computer all pertinent information, e.g., dosage of ^{18}F-FDG, injection time, and number of bed positions.
18. Position the patient to the upper limit of scan in the scanner.
19. Collect a patient's transmission scan with the ^{68}Ge source.

20. Start the patient's emission scan collecting data for a preset count or time.
21. Move the table to the next bed position and repeat steps 19 and 20. Note: Steps 19, 20 and 21 are automatically done by the computer control.
22. The scanner stops when the lower limit of the scan is completed (that is, scanning at all bed positions is completed).
23. The patient is released after the complete acquisition of the data.

Reconstruction and Storage

24. Attenuation correction factors are calculated from the blank transmission scan (Step 12) and patient transmission scan (Step 19). Reconstruct images using the corrected data with appropriate reconstruction algorithms (FBP or iterative method), provided by the manufacturer.
25. Images are sent to the workstation for display and interpretation.
26. Images are stored and archived for future use or for use in PACS, if available.

Whole-Body PET/CT Imaging with ^{18}F-FDG

Physician Directive

1. The nuclear physician evaluates the history of the patient and also asks the patient if he/she is allergic to the iodinated CT contrast agent, if it is required in the study.
2. The physician authorizes a higher dosage of ^{18}F-FDG, if needed based on the patient's weight.

Patient Preparation

3. The patient is asked to fast for 6 hours prior to scan.
4. Remove metallic items from the patient, including dentures, pants with zipper, bra, belts, bracelets, etc.
5. The patient wears a snapless gown.
6. Insert an I.V. catheter in the patient's arm for administration of ^{18}F-FDG.

Dosage Administration

7. If the patient is diabetic, check the blood glucose level. If the level is <200 mg/dl, inject ^{18}F-FDG into the patient a dosage of 0.22 mCi/kg (8.1 MBq/kg) or as prescribed by the physician. The cutoff value for glucose level varies with the institution.

8. Intravenous or oral CT contrast agents are recommended in PET/CT studies. Intravenous agents are used for all body areas except the abdomen, for which oral contrast agents are used. Oral contrast agents are normally administered 40 to 60 minutes prior to CT scanning, whereas IV contrast agents are administered 30 to 40 seconds before CT scanning.

9. The patient waits for 45 to 60 minutes after FDG administration and is instructed to remain quiet with minimal movement until the completion of the PET/CT scan.

10. The patient is asked to void prior to scanning.

Scan

11. Enter the patient's information into the computer, such as name, clinic or hospital number, birthdate, and weight as well as the dosage of ^{18}F-FDG.

12. Collect a blank CT transmission scan at the beginning of the day. It is used for subsequent patients for the day.

13. The patient lies supine on the scan table with the head toward the gantry and is positioned by laser light. The patient's arms are positioned up or down depending on the area to be scanned. Comfortable supports are provided for the head and neck, the arms and the knees.

14. The table advances by computer control toward the gantry (first CT). Acquire a topogram to define axial range of the body for scanning. The patient is asked not to move, close eyes and breathe normally during this phase. When the area to be scanned is covered by the topogram, scanning is stopped.

15. Position the patient in the CT scan field and procure a spiral CT transmission scan that takes less than 1 min. If an intravenous contrast agent is needed, inject it just 20–50 seconds prior to the CT scan is started.

16. After the completion of the CT scan, the table is automatically advanced into the PET scanner with the patient in the scan field. The number of bed positions is automatically ascertained from the axial range defined by the topogram in Step 14. Data are acquired for a set time for each bed position.

17. After the completion of the PET data acquisition for the last bed position, the patient is released.

Reconstruction and Storage

18. Because CT images are collected in a short time, they are ready for calculation of attenuation correction factors before the first PET emission scan is obtained. The attenuation correction factors are calculated from the blank scan (Step 7) and patient's tansmission scan (Step 15) by the appropriate algorithm.

19. Attenuation correction factors are applied to acquired PET data. PET images are then reconstructed from corrected data using either the FBP or the iterative method depending on the vendor's software.
20. The appropriate software fuses the CT and PET images of each slice.
21. The CT, PET, and fused PET/CT images are then sent to the workstation for display and interpretation.
22. Images are stored and archived for future use or for use in PACS, if available.

Myocardial Metabolic PET Imaging with ^{18}F-FDG

Patient Preparation

1. The patient is instructed to fast for 6 to 12 hours prior to scan.
2. Blood glucose level of the patient is checked. A variety of situations can arise as to glucose loading to titrate blood glucose level. For details, refer to the American Society of Nuclear Cardiology Practice Guidelines: PET myocardial glucose metabolism and perfusion imaging (Bacharach et al., 2003). One standard protocol is adopted as follows:
   (a) If fasting glucose level <125 mg/dL and no diabetes, then the patient is given 25 g of glucose orally.
   (b) If the fasting glucose level is between 125 and 225 mg/dL, 13 g of glucose is given orally.
   (c) For glucose level >225 mg/dL, insulin dosage units based on the formula (glucose level −50)/25 are given intravenously.
   (d) After 30 to 60 minutes, if the glucose level is yet greater than 150 mg/dL, more insulin is administered I.V. until the glucose level drops below 150 mg/dL.
3. Place an IV catheter in the arm of the patient for administration of ^{18}F- FDG.

Dosage Administration

4. After blood glucose monitoring, administer 5 to15 mCi (185–555 MBq) ^{18}F-FDG to the glucose loaded patient.
5. The patient is asked to wait for 45 to 60 minutes.

Scan

6. Enter the patient's information into the computer, such as name, clinic number, birthdate, weight and the dosage of ^{18}F-FDG.
7. Obtain a blank transmission scan with a ^{68}Ge source befor the first patient is done. This scan is used for all subsequent patients for the day.
8. The patient lies supine on the scan table with arms up away from the field of the heart.

9. Position the patient in the scanner with the heart in the axial field of view.
10. Procure a transmission scan of the patient using the rotating ^{68}Ge source.
11. Next, collect PET emission scan data for a preset time or count in a sinogram matrix. It should take about 10 to 30 minutes.

Reconstruction and Storage

12. Attenuation correction factors are caculated from the blank transmission scan (Step 7) and patient's transmission scan (Step 10) and applied to the acquired emission data. Reconstruct images using the corrected emission data by the FBP or iterative method provided by the manufacturer. The pixel size in reconstructed images should be 2 to 3mm.
13. The gating technique may be applied, if desired.
14. Images are then sent to the workstation for viewing and interpretation.
15. Next, images are stored for future use or for use in PACS, if desired.

Myocardial Perfusion PET Imaging with ^{82}Rb-RbCl

Patient Preparation

1. The patient removes all clothing above the waist and wears a slip-on gown.
2. Twelve-lead EKG connections are then applied to the patient for monitoring vital signs during stressing.
3. The patient lies supine on the scan table with arms stretched out beyond the scanner gantry. The head and neck and the arms are kept comfortable and immobile with supports.
4. Insert an I.V. catheter into the arm for ^{82}Rb and pharmacologic agent (dipyridamole or adenosine) infusion. The IV line is kept patent with saline. Patient's information is entered into the computer.

Dosage Administration and Scan

5. Collect a blank transmission scan at the beginning of the day by the ^{68}Ge source before the first patient is positioned in the PET scanner. This blank scan is used for all subsequent patients for the day.
6. Position the patient so that the heart is within the scan field.
7. Connect the ^{82}Rb generator tubing from the infusion pump (see Addendum) to the patient's catheter. A low dosage of 10 to 20mCi (370–740 MBq) ^{82}Rb is administered by the infusion pump and a scout scan is obtained to ensure the position of the heart is in the correct scan field.
8. Take a patient's transmission scan with the rotating ^{68}Ge source.

9. Administer ^{82}Rb by the infusion pump (see Addendum) for a cumulative activity of 40 to 60 mCi (1.48–2.22 GBq) for 2-D acquisition or 20
   to 40 mCi (0.74–1.48 GBq) for 3-D acquisition. Infusion should be completed in a period of maximum 30 seconds.
10. Start rest emission scan 70 to 90 seconds after the ^{82}Rb infusion for
    normal left ventricular function and about 110 to 130 seconds for
    poor ventricular function. Gated acquisition also can be performed, if
    desired.
11. Infuse the pharmacologic agent (dipyridamole at 0.57 mg/kg over 4
    minutes, or adenosine at 140 μg/kg/min for 6 minutes) using a pump,
    after the rest scan.
12. Administer ^{82}Rb by the infusion pump at the peak stress for the same
    cumulative activity as for the rest scan in Step 9.
13. Start stress emission scan at the peak stress collecting data for a preset
    count or time.
14. The patient is released after the completion of the PET scan.

Reconstruction and Storage

15. Attenuation correction factors are calculated for each pixel from the
    transmission scan (Step 8) and the blank scan (Step 5) and applied to
    the PET emission data. Reconstruct images using the corrected data by
    the FBP or iterative method based on the algorithm provided by the
    manufacturer. The reconstruction should use a Butterworth or low-pass
    filter and a pixel size of 2 to 3 mm.
16. Images are sent to the workstation for display and interpretation.
17. Images are stored and archived for future use or for use in PACS, if
    desired.

Addendum

^{82}Rb Infusion Pump

Rubidium-82 ($t_{1/2}$ = 75 seconds) is available from the ^{82}Sr-^{82}Rb generator
(supplied by Bracco Diagnostics, Inc.). Because of its short half-life, an automated infusion pump is employed for its delivery from the generator to the
patient. The infusion pump is a device manufactured by RbM Services and
distributed by Bracco Diagnostics Inc. that delivers ^{82}Rb by pumping 0.9%
NaCl (normal saline) through the generator. A schematic diagram of the
infusion pump is shown in Figure 11-1. The lead-shielded generator is
mounted on a mobile cart. A large-volume plastic syringe is connected
through a 3-way stopcock to a saline bottle or bag to supply saline to the
generator for ^{82}Rb elution. The syringe is filled with saline and then pushes
it through the generator to elute ^{82}Rb under the action of an electronically

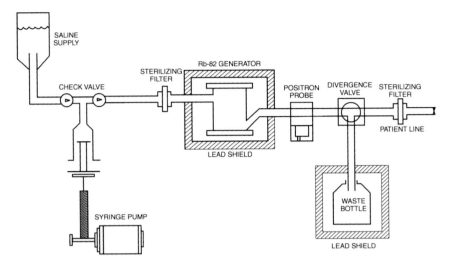

FIGURE 11-1. A schematic illustration of the ^{82}Rb infusion pump. The details of the operation of the pump are given in the text.

controlled pump. An outlet tubing from the generator carries the ^{82}Rb activity in saline under the action of the pump to either a waste bottle or the patient. A divergence valve placed along the outlet tubing switches the line between the patient and the waste bottle. The initial low-level activity is discarded into the waste bottle, and later the uniform activity is directed to the patient. In the midway of the tubing before the divergence valve, a positron detector made of plastic scintillator coupled with a photomultiplier tube is installed to measure the activity passing through the tubing.

The infusion pump is operated electronically and equipped with several controls on a console that select the total volume (ml), total dosage (mCi), dosage rate (mCi/s), and flow rate (ml/min). A printer is included in the device to print out all parameters related to the infusion of the ^{82}Rb activity. Before the infusion pump is used for a given day, the pump device needs to be calibrated. There is a control knob on the console that sets a specified calibration factor for the generator. Calibration is performed at the beginning of the day prior to patient study using the calibration factor given for the generator. After flushing the low activity volume, the ^{82}Rb activity is collected in a vial for a certain time and measured in a dose calibrator immediately after the infusion is over. The measured activity is corrected for decay to the end of infusion and compared with the activity printed out by the printer. The discrepancy, beyond the specifications of the manufacturer, is corrected by adjusting the calibration factor and repeating the calibration. In this calibration experiment, the amounts of ^{82}Sr ($t_{1/2} = 25.6$ days) and ^{85}Sr ($t_{1/2} = 65$ days) breakthrough are also determined by allowing the

[82]Rb activity in the vial to decay completely and then measuring the activity of these two radionuclides, which must be within the limit set by the manufacturer.

For a patient study, the patient gets an IV catheter that is connected to the patient line of the infusion pump. The desired total volume, total activity to be administered and the flow rate are all set on the console by the operator prior to the start of infusion. First, the low activity volume of saline as detected by the detector is flushed out to the waste bottle by applying the purge button. After purging, when the preset dose rate threshold is achieved as detected by the detector, the activity is directed to the patient line, and the set amount of the cumulated activity is administered. The pump stops after the infusion of the desired amount of activity, and all relevant parameters are printed out by the printer.

The waste bottle should be emptied every morning prior to or at the end of system usage. The [82]Rb generator is supplied once a month, which is installed in the infusion cart replacing the old generator. Each new generator is supplied with a new tubing set (called the administration set), which replaces the old set. The old generator is returned to the supplier, Bracco Diagnostics, Inc.

Reference and Suggested Reading

1. Bacharach SL, Bax JJ, Case J, et al. PET myocardial glucose metabolism and perfusion imaging. Part 1. Guidelines for patient preparation and data acquisition. *J Nucl Cardiol.* 2003;10:543.

Appendix A
Abbreviations Used in the Text

ALARA	as low as reasonably achievable
ANDA	abbreviated new drug application
APC	ambulatory payment classification
BGO	bismuth germanate
CMS	Centers for Medicare and Medicaid Services
CPT	Current Procedural Terminology
DAC	derived air concentration
DICOM	Digital Imaging and Communications in Medicine
DOT	Department of Transportation
DRG	Diagnosis Related Group
EC	electron capture
FBP	filtered backprojection
FDA	Food and Drug Administration
FDG	fluorodeoxyglucose
FOV	field of view
GSO	gadolinium oxyorthosilicate
HCPCS	Healthcare Common Procedure Coding System
HIPAA	Hospital Insurance Portability and Accountability Act
HIS	Hospital Information System
HOPPS	Hospital Outpatient Prospective Payment System
HVL	half-value layer
ICD-9-CM	International Classification of Disease, Ninth Revision, Clinical Modification
ICRP	International Committee on Radiological Protection
IND	Notice of Claimed Investigational Exemption for a New Drug
IRB	Institutional Review Board
IT	isomeric transition
kV	kilovolt
LAN	local area network
LCD	liquid crystal display
LOR	line of response
LSO	lutetium oxyorthosilicate

MIRD	medical internal radiation dose
MLEM	maximum-likelihood expectation maximization
NCA	no carrier added
NCD	national coverage determination
NCRP	National Council on Radiation Protection and Measurement
NDA	New Drug Application
NECR	noise equivalent count rate
NEMA	National Electrical Manufacturers Association
NRC	Nuclear Regulatory Commission
OSEM	ordered subset expectation maximization
PACS	Picture Archival and Communication System
PET	positron emission tomography
PM	photomultiplier (tube)
PHA	pulse height analyzer
QF	quality factor
RBE	relative biologic effectiveness
RDRC	Radioactive Drug Research Committee
RIS	Radiology Information System
RSC	Radiation Safety Committee
RSO	Radiation Safety Officer
RVU	relative value unit
SF	scatter fraction
SPECT	single photon emission computed tomography
SUV	standard uptake value
TEDE	total effective dose equivalent
TLC	thin layer chromatography
TLD	thermoluminescent dosimeter
USP	US Pharmacopeia

Appendix B
Terms Used in the Text

Absorption. A process by which the total energy of a radiation is removed by a medium through which it passes.

Annihilation radiation. Gamma radiations of 511 keV energy emitted at 180° after a β^+ particle is annihilated by combining with an electron in matter.

Atomic mass unit (amu). By definition, one-twelfth of the mass of ^{12}C, equal to 1.66×10^{-24} g or 931 MeV.

Atomic number (Z). The number of protons in the nucleus of an atom.

Attenuation. A process by which the intensity of radiation is reduced by absorption and/or scattering during its passage through matter.

Auger electron. An electron ejected from the outer electron shell by an x-ray by transferring all its energy.

Average life (τ). See Mean life.

Avogadro's number. The number of molecules in 1 g·mole of a substance, or the number of atoms in 1 g·atom of an element. It is equal to 6.02×10^{23}.

Becquerel (Bq). A unit of radioactivity. One becquerel is equal to 1 disintegration per second.

Binding energy. The energy to bind 2 entities together. In a nucleus, it is the energy needed to separate a nucleon from other nucleons in the nucleus. In a chemical bond, it is the energy necessary to separate two binding partners by an infinite distance.

Biological half-life (T_b). The time by which one-half of an administered dosage of a substance is eliminated by biological processes such as urinary and fecal excretion.

Bremsstrahlung. Gamma-ray photons produced by deceleration of charged particles near the nucleus of an atom.

Carrier. A stable element that is added in detectable quantities to a radionuclide of the same element, usually to facilitate chemical processing of the radionuclide.

Carrier-free. A term used to indicate the absence of any stable isotopic atom in a radionuclide sample.

Chelating agent. A compound that binds to a metal ion by more than one coordinate covalent bond.

Committed dose equivalent ($H_{T,50}$). The dose equivalent to organs or tissues of reference (T) that will be received from an intake of radioactive material by an individual during the 50-year period following intake.

Conversion electron (e^-). *See* Internal conversion.

Cross section (σ). The probability of occurrence of a nuclear reaction or the formation of a radionuclide in a nuclear reaction. It is expressed in a unit termed barn; 1 barn = 10^{-24} cm^2.

Curie (Ci). A unit of activity. A curie is defined as 3.7×10^{10} disintegrations per second.

Cyclotron. A machine to accelerate charged particles in circular paths by means of an electromagnetic field. The accelerated particles such as α particles, protons, deuterons, and heavy ions possess high energies and can cause nuclear reactions in target atoms by irradiation.

Decay constant (λ). The fraction of atoms of a radioactive element decaying per unit time. It is expressed as $\lambda = 0.693/t_{1/2}$ where $t_{1/2}$ is the half-life of the radionuclide.

Deep-dose equivalent (H_d). Dose equivalent at a tissue depth of 1 cm (1000 mg/cm^2) due to external whole body exposure.

Dosage. A general term for the amount of a radiopharmaceutical administered in microcuries or millicuries, or becquerels.

Dose. The energy of radiation absorbed by any matter.

Dosimeter. An instrument to measure the cumulative dose of radiation received during a period of radiation exposure.

Dosimetry. The calculation or measurement of radiation absorbed doses.

Effective dose (H_E). An estimated whole-body dose weighted for radiosensitivity of each organ. It is calculated by summing the product of dose equivalent (H_r) and tissue radiosensitivity (W_T) of each organ, $\sum_{T,r} H_{T,r} \cdot W_T$.

Effective half-life (T_e). Time required for an initial administered dose to be reduced to one half due to both physical decay and biological elimination of a radionuclide. It is given by $T_e = (T_p \times T_b)/(T_p + T_b)$, where T_e is the effective half-life, and T_p and T_b are the physical and biological half-lives, respectively.

Electron (e^-). A negatively charged particle circulating around the atomic nucleus. It has a charge of 4.8×10^{-10} electrostatic units and a mass of 9.1×10^{-28} g, equivalent to 0.511 MeV, or equal to 1/1836 of the mass of a proton.

Electron capture (EC). A mode of decay of a proton-rich radionuclide in which an orbital electron is captured by the nucleus, accompanied by emission of a neutrino and characteristic x-rays.

Electron volt (eV). The kinetic energy gained by an electron when accelerated through a potential difference of 1 volt.

Erg. The unit of energy or work done by a force of 1 dyne through a distance of 1 cm.

Fission (*f*). A nuclear process by which a heavy nucleus divides into two nearly equal smaller nuclei, along with the emission of 2 to 3 neutrons.

Generator, radionuclide. A device in which a short-lived daughter nuclide is separated chemically from a long-lived parent nuclide adsorbed on an adsorbent material. For example, ^{99m}Tc is separated from ^{99}Mo from the ^{99}Mo-^{99m}Tc generator with saline.

Gray (*Gy*). The unit of radiation dose in SI units. One gray is equal to 100 rad.

Half-life ($t_{1/2}$). A unique characteristic of a radionuclide, defined by the time during which an initial activity of a radionuclide is reduced to one half. It is related to the decay constant λ by $t_{1/2} = 0.693/\lambda$.

Half-value layer (*HVL*). The thickness of an absorbing material required to reduce the intensity or exposure of a radiation beam to one-half of the initial value when placed in the path of the beam.

Internal conversion. An alternative mode to γ-ray decay in which nuclear excitation energy is transferred to an orbital electron which is then ejected from the orbit.

Ion. An atom or group of atoms with a positive charge (cation) or a negative charge (anion).

Ionization chamber. A gas-filled instrument used to measure radioactivity or exposure in terms of ion pairs produced in gas by radiations.

Isobars. Nuclides having the same mass number, that is, the same total number of neutrons and protons. Examples are $^{57}_{26}$Fe and $^{57}_{27}$Co.

Isomeric transition (IT). Decay of the excited state of a nuclide to another lower excited state or the ground state.

Isomers. Nuclides having the same atomic and mass numbers but differing in energy and spin of the nuclei. For example, ^{99}Tc and ^{99m}Tc are isomers.

Isotones. Nuclides have the same number of neutrons in the nucleus. For example, $^{131}_{53}$I and $^{132}_{54}$Xe are isotones.

Isotopes. Nuclides having the same atomic number, that is, the same number of protons in the nucleus. Examples are $^{14}_{6}$C and $^{12}_{6}$C.

K capture. A mode of radioactive decay in which an electron from the K shell is captured by the nucleus.

$LD_{50/60}$. A dosage of a substance that, when administered or applied to a group of any living species, kills 50% of the group in 60 days.

Linear attenuation coefficient (μ). The fraction of radiation energy absorbed and scattered per unit thickness of absorber.

Linear energy transfer (*LET*). Energy deposited by radiation per unit length of the matter through which the radiation passes. Its usual unit is keV/μm.

Mass number (*A*). The total number of protons and neutrons in a nucleus of a nuclide.

Mean life (τ). The period of time a radionuclide exists on the average before disintegration. It is related to the half-life and decay constant by $\tau = 1/\lambda = 1.44t_{1/2}$.

Metastable state (*m*). An excited state of a nuclide that decays to another excited state or the ground state with a measurable half-life.

Neutrino (v). A particle of no charge and mass emitted with variable energy during β^+ and electron capture decays of radionuclides.

No carrier added (NCA). A term used to characterize the state of a radioactive material to which no stable isotope of the compound has been added purposely.

Nucleon. A common term for neutrons or protons in the nucleus of a nuclide.

pH. The unit of hydrogen ion concentration. It is given by the negative common logarithm of the hydrogen ion concentration in a solution: $pH = -\log_{10} [H^+]$.

Phantom. A volume of material artificially made to simulate the property of an organ or part of the body when exposed to radiation.

Physical half-life (T_p). *See* Half-life.

Quality factor (*QF*). A factor dependent on linear energy transfer that is multiplied by absorbed doses to calculate the dose equivalents in rem. It is used in radiation protection in order to take into account the relative radiation damage caused by different radiations. It is 1 for x, γ, and β rays, 10 for neutrons and protons, and 20 for α particles.

Rad. The unit of radiation absorbed dose. One rad is equal to 100 ergs of radiation energy deposited per gram of any matter, or 10^{-2} J/kg of any medium.

Radiation weighting factor (W_r). See Quality factor.

Radiochemical purity. The fraction of the total radioactivity in the desired chemical form. If ^{99m}Tc-MAA Is 90% pure, then 90% of the radioactivity is in the ^{99M}Tc-MAA form.

Radionuclidic purity. The fraction of the total radioactivity in the form of the stated radionuclide. Any extraneous radioactivity such as ^{99}Mo in ^{99m}Tc-radiopharmaceuticals is an impurity.

Radiopharmaceutical. A radioactive drug that can be administered safely to humans for diagnostic and therapeutic purposes.

Rem. A dose equivalent defined by the absorbed dose (rad) times the relative biological effectiveness or quality factor or radiation weighting factor of the radiation in question.

Roentgen. The quantity of x-rays or γ radiations that produces one electrostatic unit of positive or negative charge in 1 cm^3 of air at 0°C and 760 mm Hg pressure (STP). It is equal to 2.58×10^{-4} C/kg air.

Sensitivity. The number of counts per unit time detected by a scanner for each unit of activity present in a source. It is given by counts per second per microcurie (cps/μCi) or (cps/MBq).

Shallow-dose equivalent (H_s). Dose equivalent at a tissue depth of 0.007cm ($7\,mg/cm^2$) averaged over an area of $1\,cm^2$ due to external exposure to the skin.

Sievert (*Sv*). The unit of dose equivalent and equal to 100rem.

Spatial resolution. A measure of the ability of a scanner to faithfully reproduce the image of an object.

Tissue weighting factor (W_T). A factor related to the radiosensitivity of different tissues in living systems.

Tracer. A radionuclide or a compound labeled with a radionuclide that may be used to follow its distribution or course through a chemical, physical, or metabolic process.

Appendix C
Units and Constants

Energy

1 electron volt (eV)	=	1.602×10^{-12} erg
1 kiloelectron volt (keV)	=	1.602×10^{-9} erg
1 million electron volts (MeV)	=	1.602×10^{-6} erg
1 joule (J)	=	10^{7} ergs
1 watt (W)	=	10^{7} ergs/s
	=	1 J/s
1 rad	=	1×10^{-2} J/kg
	=	100 ergs/g
1 gray (Gy)	=	100 rad
	=	1 J/kg
1 sievert (Sv)	=	100 rem
	=	1 J/kg
1 horsepower (HP)	=	746 W
1 calorie (cal)	=	4.184 J

Charge

1 coulomb (C)	=	6.25×10^{18} charges
1 electronic charge	=	4.8×10^{-10} electrostatic unit
	=	1.6×10^{-19} C
1 ampere (A)	=	1 C/s

Mass and Energy

1 atomic mass unit (amu)	=	1.66×10^{-24} g
	=	1/12 the atomic weight of ^{12}C
	=	931 MeV
1 electron rest mass	=	0.511 MeV
1 proton rest mass	=	938.78 MeV
1 neutron rest mass	=	939.07 MeV
1 pound	=	453.6 g

Length

1 angstrom (Å)	=	10^{-8} cm
1 micrometer or micron (μm)	=	10^{-6} meter
	=	10^4 Å
1 nanometer (nm)	=	10^{-9} meter
1 fermi (F)	=	10^{-13} cm
1 inch	=	2.54 cm

Activity

1 curie (Ci)	=	3.7×10^{10} disintegrations per second (dps)
	=	2.22×10^{12} disintegrations per minute (dpm)
1 millicurie (mCi)	=	3.7×10^7 dps
	=	2.22×10^9 dpm
1 microcurie (μCi)	=	3.7×10^4 dps
	=	2.22×10^6 dpm
1 becquerel (Bq)	=	1 dps
	=	2.703×10^{-11} Ci
1 kilobecquerel (kBq)	=	10^3 dps
	=	2.703×10^{-8} Ci
1 megabecquerel (MBq)	=	10^6 dps
	=	2.703×10^{-5} Ci
1 gigabecquerel (GBq)	=	10^9 dps
	=	2.703×10^{-2} Ci
1 terabecquerel (TBq)	=	10^{12} dps
	=	27.03 Ci

Constants

Avogadro's number	=	6.02×10^{23} atoms/g·atom
	=	6.02×10^{23} molecules/g·mole
π	=	3.1416
e	=	2.7183

Appendix D
Estimated Absorbed Doses from Intravenous Administration of ^{18}F-FDG and ^{82}Rb-RbCl

The dose estimate D in each organ is made by using the following internal dosimetry equation:

$$D = \tilde{A} \cdot S$$

where $\tilde{A}$ is the cumulated activity and S is the mean absorbed dose per cumulated activity. $\tilde{A}$ is calculated from the initial administered activity and the biodistribution and residence time of the tracer in each organ. S is calculated from the knowledge of physical characteristics of the radiation in question, the mass of the organ and the absorption fraction of the radiation in the target organ. The values of S are available in literature for most common radiopharmaceuticals including ^{18}F-FDG. The experimental data for biodistribution and residence time are available in literature and used to calculate $\tilde{A}$. The following two tables give the absorbed doses per unit administered activity based on these calculations for ^{18}F-FDG and ^{82}Rb-RbCl, respectively.

Absorbed dose per unit administered activity of ^{18}F-FDG[1]

Target organ	mGy/MBq	rad/mCi
Brain	0.046 ± 0.012	0.17 ± 0.044
Heart wall	0.068 ± 0.036	0.25 ± 0.13
Kidneys	0.021 ± 0.0059	0.078 ± 0.022
Liver	0.024 ± 0.0085	0.088 ± 0.031
Lungs	0.015 ± 0.0084	0.056 ± 0.031
Pancreas	0.014 ± 0.0016	0.052 ± 0.0060
Red marrow	0.011 ± 0.0017	0.040 ± 0.0062
Spleen	0.015 ± 0.0021	0.056 ± 0.0078
Urinary bladder wall[2]	0.073 ± 0.042	0.27 ± 0.16
Ovaries[3]	0.011 ± 0.0015	0.041 ± 0.0055
Testes[3]	0.011 ± 0.0016	0.041 ± 0.0057
Whole Body[5]	0.012 ± 0.00077	0.043 ± 0.0023
Effective dose[4,5]	0.070	0.019

[1] Reproduced with permission from Hays MT, Watson EE, Thomas ER, et al. MIRD Dose Estimate Report No. 19: Radiation Absorbed Dose Estimates from ^{18}F-FDG. *J Nucl Med.* 2002;43:210.

[2] Dose to urinary bladder wall is based on 120-min void intervals, starting 120min after dosing, using traditional static MIRD model.

[3] Doses to ovaries and testes include doses from residence times in urinary bladder and remainder of body as calculated from data in: Hays and Segall. A mathematical model for the distribution of fluorodeoxyglucose in humans. *J Nucl Med.* 1999;40:1358.

[4] From ICRP Publication No. 80. New York: Pergamon Press; 1999.

[5] The calculation of whole body dose is based on total energy deposited in the body divided by its total mass, whereas the total effective dose reported by ICRP is calculated by applying risk-based weighting factors to individual organ doses to estimate a uniform whole-body dose that in theory gives the same risk as the non-uniform pattern that actually occurred. The two values are based on different concepts and not comparable.

Absorbed dose per unit administered activity of ^{82}Rb-RbCl[1]

Target organ	μGy/MBq	mrad/mCi
Heart wall	1.90	7.03
Kidneys	8.60	31.83
Liver	0.86	3.18
Lungs	1.70	6.28
Small intestine	1.4	5.18
Stomach	0.86	3.18
Testes	0.30	1.12
Whole body	0.43	1.58
Effective dose[2]	3.40	12.58

[1] Obtained from package insert.

[2] Obtained from ICRP Publication No. 80, New York: Pergamon Press, 1999.

Appendix E
Evaluation of Tumor Uptake of ^{18}F-FDG by PET

PET imaging is widely used for the detection of a variety of tumors such as breast, colorectal, esophageal, head and neck, lung, thyroid, melanoma, lymphoma, and other cancers, because of its high sensitivity, specificity, and accuracy. In the interpretation of tumor FDG-PET images, it is desirable to compare the relative tumor FDG uptake with the adjacent normal tissue uptake. Such a comparison offers information on the degree of tumor progression and provides clues to appropriate management of the tumor. In radiation therapy or chemotherapy of tumors, comparative evaluation of tumor FDG-PET images before and after therapy is even more useful to assess the effect of therapy on tumor. In all cases the reconstructed images are used to determine the tumor uptake of FDG relative to the normal tissue uptake.

There are several methods, visual, quantitative, and semi-quantitative, to determine the tumor uptake of FDG. Visual assessment is commonly used in tumor diagnosis and staging, and is based on differences in contrast between tumor and adjacent tissue. This is a simplified method requiring only a single static image at a set time after injection and can be equally applied to assess the therapeutic response of the tumor. In the visual technique, it is important to adjust the image intensities of the tumor and adjacent tissues to the same gray or color scale.

While visual assessment of tumor is widely accepted in many nuclear medicine facilities, the quantitative or even semiquantitative method improves the detection and comparative assessment significantly and therefore is highly desirable. Quantitative methods, also called the kinetic methods, include two methods: compartmental analysis and Potlak analysis. Compartmental analysis is based on the fitting of the time-activity curve to a two-compartmental model, using measured arterial activity (input function) and non-linear regression. The time course of activity in tissue is followed by serial imaging and arterial blood sampling. The metabolic rate of glucose given by this method is expressed in moles/min/ml. Potlak analysis provides similar information requiring a fewer data and only the integral of the blood activity for input function. Both methods are too complex and demanding of resources, and therefore are less favorable for routine clinical application. The details of these methods are beyond the scope of this book and the readers are referred to standard texts on kinetic modeling.

In semiquantitative methods, static images are utilized as in visual assessment to determine the tissue activity and compare the relative tumor uptake. One method uses an index, the tumor-to-normal tissue activity ratio (T/N), using data from the normal and tumor regions on the reconstructed images. The ratios are independent of the administered dosage, patient's weight or blood glucose level. The T/N ratio assessment is somewhat similar to visual assessment. The choice of an appropriate normal reference site, particularly in the abdomen and pelvic area, is critical in this analysis.

The most versatile semiquantitative technique is the *standard uptake value* (SUV) method that is widely used in nuclear medicine and molecular imaging. This value is also less commonly referred to as the differential uptake ratio (DUR). It is defined by the tissue concentration of activity as determined from the region of interest (ROI) on the PET image, divided by the injected dosage of the tracer, and multiplied by a calibration factor, which is basically the body weight, body surface or body lean mass. Thus,

$$SUV = (C_{ROI}/A) \times WT \tag{E.1}$$

where C_{ROI} is the decay corrected radiotracer concentration in μCi/g(Bq/g) of tissue in ROI, A is the injected radiotracer dosage in μCi(Bq), and WT is the body weight of the patient. In SUV calculation, an ROI is chosen by the reader on the reconstructed image that is displayed on the computer monitor. The computer then calculates the average count density or maximum count density in the ROI, correct it for the decay for the uptake period and counting efficiency, estimates the area of ROI from the knowledge of pixel size and the number of pixels in ROI, and finally converts the corrected count density to activity per gram of tissue (assuming tissue density is equal to 1 g/cc). From the knowledge of the body weight of the patient, and the injected dosage in μCi(Bq), the SUV is calculated for the ROI using Eq. (E.1). The FDG SUV values are unitless numbers, and for some normal tissues are: <1 for soft tissues; 1.5 to 2.0 for blood pool 1 hour after injection; ~2.5 for liver and ~3.5 for renal cortex. The SUV values for various neoplastic tissues range from 2 to as high as 25, depending on the avidity of the different cancer cells for FDG. Note that if all of the tracer were uniformly distributed throughout the body, the SUV in each region would be 1. It implies that the SUV serves as a normalized T/N ratio index.

It is important to note that the SUV values are affected by several factors. The time period between tracer injection and scanning (i.e., the uptake period) is perhaps the largest single source of error in determining the SUV. Time to reach maximum uptake in a given tissue varies with the type and condition of tissue i.e., different forms of neoplasm and also with tissues before and after therapy. Tissue uptake of FDG decreases with increasing blood glucose level, which affects the SUV. Excess body fat falsely elevates the SUV, which many investigators correct by using body lean mass instead of body weight. Also, many investigators found better values of SUVs using body surface area in place of body weight. The use of maximum pixel count density versus average value for all pixels in an ROI also affects the SUV values, although the average value now is less commonly used. Thus, SUVs reported in literature are not exactly comparable unless all these parameters are specified.

Appendix F
Answers to Questions

Chapter 1
5. false
6. true
11. 85 keV
14. 110 keV
16. 220 min
18. 4.6 mCi
19. 31.1 mCi
20. 1.56 hr
21. 1.55 hr
23. (a) false, (b) false, (c) true
25. (a) false, (b) true
26. 325 keV
29. (a) 8.3 HVLs, (b) 9 HVLs
31. 2.56 cm

Chapter 2
11. (a) true, (b) false, (c) true
12. 120 cm

Chapter 3
2. (a)
3. (b)
5. true
11. true
13. 0.135
15. true

Chapter 4
6. 3.15 mm
11. true

Chapter 5
3. false
4. true
5. 8 mm
7. 1.98 mm
10. C
12. 2-D: (b); 3-D: (a)
13. C
17. true
18. A. true, B. false
19. B

Chapter 6
5. true
6. 3.86 Ci
7. ~18 hr (6 half-lives of the radionuclide)
9. true

Chapter 7
10. false

Chapter 8
3. false
19. 9.76 mR
20. 2.61 cm
21. 10%
24. true

Chapter 10
3. 1.94 cm of lead
(assuming occupancy factor = 1)

Index